Technology, Health Care, and Management in the Hospital of the Future

EDITED BY Eliezer Geisler,
Koos Krabbendam,
AND Roel Schuring

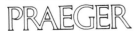

Westport, Connecticut
London

64.95

Library of Congress Cataloging-in-Publication Data

Technology, health care, and management in the hospital of the future / edited by
Eliezer Geisler, Koos Krabbendam, Roel Schuring.
    p. cm.
    Includes bibliographical references and index.
    ISBN 1–56720–623–9 (alk. paper)
    1. Hospitals—Technological innovations—Congresses. 2. Medical care—
Technological innovations—Congresses. 3. Hospitals—Administration—
Congresses. 4. Medical innovations—Congresses. 5. Technological innovations—
Congresses. I. Geisler, Eliezer, 1942– II. Krabbendam, Koos. III. Schuring, Roel.
    RA971.6.T43 2003
    362.1'1'068—dc21   2002029875

British Library Cataloguing in Publication Data is available.

Library of Congress Catalog Card Number: 2002029875
ISBN: 1–56720–623–9

First published in 2003

Praeger Publishers, 88 Post Road West, Westport, CT 06881
An imprint of Greenwood Publishing Group, Inc.
www.praeger.com

Printed in the United States of America

The paper used in this book complies with the
Permanent Paper Standard issued by the National
Information Standards Organization (Z39.48–1984).

10 9 8 7 6 5 4 3 2 1

03-04-929 BT

Contents

Acknowledgments

The editors wish to thank the authors for their insightful ideas and research that peers into the future of technology and management in healthcare delivery. We also thank the faculty and staff at the University of Twente for hosting the First International Conference on the Hospital of the Future, thus permitting us a forum for the authors to present their work. We thank all the organizations that supported the conference and the many scholars and practitioners who attended it. We are grateful to Praeger Publishers; to our production editor, John Donohue; and especially to Dr. Janet Goranson, who assisted us in the preparation of the manuscript; we are very appreciative of her professional advice and expertise. Finally, we are deeply obliged to our families, who supported us in the effort of making this book a reality.

About This Book

As the twenty-first century unfolds, major transformations are occurring in the delivery of health care worldwide. Medical and healthcare technologies are increasingly impacting the clinical and the administrative dimensions of healthcare delivery. Innovations introduced in the 1990s have already created accumulated effects that will be compounded by the continuous technological progress in medical care. Areas such as telemedicine, telehealth, computerized medical records, and uses of the Internet are some of the milestones in the almost total revamping of the healthcare landscape.

A key ingredient in this age of challenges and transformations is the redesign of the hospital as a provider of medical care. Medical technology is already changing the operations, mission, and processes of today's hospitals. In this regard, the challenges for the future represent an exciting opportunity for study, reflection, planning, and intervention.

This book is a compilation of selected papers presented at the First International Conference on the Hospital of the Future held at the University of Twente, the Netherlands, in April 2001. Over 100 academics and practitioners from 14 countries presented exciting papers that described recent developments in the technological transformations of the sector of healthcare delivery.

The purpose of this book is to offer to the reader this exciting and timely set of papers in a format that constitutes a cohesive description of key elements of the hospital of the future. The papers are the outcome of the four main themes or tracks of the conference. These themes were:

1. *Changes and Transformations in Society.* What will be the changes that occur in societal attitudes toward health care and medical care? How will these changes impact the hospital of the future? What will be the changes in behavioral patterns concerning the role that technology plays in healthcare delivery? What will be the changes in the needs and expressed desires of customers, regulators, and providers in the new era of medical technology and the ubiquity of the Internet?

2. *Applications of Information Technologies.* How will uses of telemedicine, telehealth, electronic applications of data and information, and electronic medical records affect healthcare delivery. What are the organizational and economics issues and challenges? How can we resolve them? How will they impact and shape the hospital of the future?

3. *Emerging Technologies.* How will new developments in technology contribute to medical care, the hospital of the future, and healthcare delivery? What are the uses and challenges of gene therapies and genetic technologies, imaging technologies, and the combined effects of joint applications of diverse technologies in healthcare delivery?

4. *Applications of Modern Management.* How will applications of modern management techniques such as total quality management, the electronic patient record, continuous improvements, and organizational restructuring contribute to the efficiency of the hospital of the future and improved healthcare delivery?

AUDIENCES

This book is geared toward the following audiences:

1. Professionals and practitioners in healthcare delivery management. These include hospital administrators, physicians, nurses, physician-assistants, and people involved with setting policies in healthcare delivery.

2. Researchers, professors, and students in the broad areas of healthcare management in universities and colleges, and scholars and other academics in the area of technology management.

3. Managers and practitioners in industrial companies that make, sell, and maintain medical equipment, medical instruments, and other medical technology.

4. Managers and other interested parties in the financial and regulatory aspects of healthcare delivery, such as insurance companies, government agencies (the Health Care Finance Administration, the National Institutes of Health, and the Food and Drug Administration), and state and local agencies.

5. The public at large who are interested in the topic of the hospital of the future—since we are all patients of healthcare delivery at some points in our lives.

In summary, the audiences for this book are the professionals and academics in healthcare management and healthcare technology management. They come from universities, industrial companies, insurance companies (payors), and government agencies. All these audiences will benefit from learning about trends and directions in the hospital of the future.

OUTLINE OF THE BOOK

This book is divided into three parts: "Creating Frameworks," "Future Processes of Healthcare Delivery," and "Emerging Technologies: Adoption, Adaptation, and Implementation." Part I contains chapters that describe organizational changes in future healthcare delivery; Part II examines different processes of delivery, such as strategic planning, palliative care, and the impact of research knowledge; Part III has chapters that address emerging technologies and their potential impacts on future care.

STRENGTHS AND UNIQUENESS

This book offers an international view across countries and a diversity of healthcare delivery systems. It includes contributions from the United States, Europe, Japan, and Australia.

The book is unique in that it concentrates on the hospital (and its variants in healthcare delivery) as the focal point for new developments in health care. The breadth of contributions and the variety of topic make this book an exciting assembly of the culmination of ongoing research that spans over a decade of scholarship.

We believe that the twenty-first century, heralded by many as the "Century of Biology," will indeed induce many revolutionary transformations in how health care and medicine are practiced and delivered. Impacts of technological breakthroughs in electronics, information, and bioengineering will create new scenarios and new realities for providers, patients, payors, and regulators.

This book is an initial step in the arduous task of identifying trends of such future transformations. We trust that the reader will be challenged by the contributions and the ideas they contain.

The Hospital of the Future: Concepts and Directions

Eliezer Geisler and Pieter Vierhout

The delivery of health care has become a worldwide area of national concern. Regardless of the system used to pay for it, healthcare delivery has constantly become more complex and more expensive. American healthcare delivery has over 7,000 hospitals and consumes one-sixth of the gross national product. A key element in the making of healthcare delivery is the role played by medical technology.

As we peer into the future, what will be the state of healthcare delivery, and what role will technology play in such scenarios? Which current trends will continue in the coming years? Which will intensify? And will healthcare delivery be subjected to the foreseeable changes in the economy and society?

KEY TRENDS

Healthcare delivery organizations are notoriously ineffective in adopting and applying new technologies. But they ultimately tend to utilize innovations in both the clinical and managerial aspects of their existence.

In the past decade we have witnessed four key trends that seem to have shaped the present and the future of healthcare delivery organizations. Although manifested primarily in the United States, these trends can now be seen in the European Union, Canada, and other countries. These trends are: (1) cost containment, (2) integration and alliances, (3) information and telecommunication, and (4) adoption of breakthrough innovations.

COST CONTAINMENT

Under the aura of managed care, capitation, and similar terms, health-care providers have applied a variety of technological innovations that have impacted both the clinical and administrative aspects of delivery of medical services. For example, innovations in orthoscopic surgery have generated a dramatic increase in outpatient versus inpatient admissions, characterized by shorter operations with local anesthesia and the ability to discharge patients as soon as a few hours after the operation. This emphasis on cost-cutting and cost-saving operations and procedures has provided incentives to practitioners and the industry to move toward standardization in medical and administrative workflows, efficiencies in purchasing and usage, and the promotion of cooperative efforts among providers.

Cost containment became the guidepost for the various payors, inasmuch as it dictated their policies and decision making. In the United States, federal and state payors of Medicare and Medicaid have continually imposed cost-cutting measures, aligned with pressures on providers to standardize and offer less expensive treatments whenever a choice was medically feasible. Private insurers behaved likewise, leading to an accepted "mantra" of the industry in the form of "managed care" and "cost containment."

We believe that the pressure to manage the costs of delivery will continue into the foreseeable future. Costs of health care continue to rise dangerously in the United States, despite the major restructuring of managed care in the 1990s. This trend will force providers to innovate for cost efficiencies and to continually reassess their clinical and administrative processes. Technology will play a crucial role in any further cost reductions, particularly in the implementation of telehealth and other emerging technologies. However, the medical focus alone will not suffice, as providers will have to also accelerate their organizational and structural efforts to become more efficient. Technology will be the catalyst allowing providers to fine-tune and improve all other efforts.

INTEGRATION AND ALLIANCES

Prime examples of the structural revolution that is occurring in American healthcare delivery are the mergers, integration, and strategic alliances among providers. In order to achieve efficiencies in the uses of technology and in administrative functions, mostly due to pressures from payors, providers have created a variety of cooperative arrangements. This trend is likely to continue in the foreseeable future.

Integration and other structural revolutions have also occurred in many European healthcare environments. In the Netherlands and in the

United Kingdom there has been a gradual, albeit small, change from the "cradle to grave" philosophy to a more cost-conscious format of delivery.

Medical and healthcare technologies are so intricately woven into these structural developments that adoption of technological innovations are being considered by providers on the basis of existing and proposed alliances and other changes. Technologies such as computerized medical records and the creation and maintenance of large databases are conducive to cooperative and networking efforts. Rural as well as urban providers will increasingly find it necessary to cooperate with each other in order to fully and currently partake of the application of new technologies.

INFORMATION AND TELECOMMUNICATION TECHNOLOGIES

As the twenty-first century unfolds, the three revolutions in health care—economic, structural, and technological—are converging to form an unmistaken trend of growth and transformation. The economic and structural changes will continue but will be deeply influenced by technological development. In particular, we will see the larger scale implementation of information and telecommunication technologies.

The healthcare delivery sector has been relatively slower than other industries in capturing the immense capabilities of information technology. Although there has been progress in telemedicine and similar areas, a visit to any hospital in the United States, Europe, or Asia clearly shows the gap between what the information technology industry predicts for healthcare applications of their products and what is currently utilized by providers. Industry planners boast of computerized records and connectivity and accessibility of records across hospital wards and across facilities as well as easy manipulation of substantial databases at the fingertips of providers. The current reality is much more prosaic, with caregivers who are slowly mastering the information technologies of a decade ago.

But all of this is changing, and in the coming years there will be a much more intensive implementation of information and telecommunication technology—in the form of devices, processes, and knowledge systems that will be continually and seamlessly applied across all activities of healthcare delivery. This trend is already visible in such areas as home care. The economies of home care are so dramatic (estimated at roughly half or less as expensive as traditional hospital care) that information and telecommunication technologies will be increasingly applied to in situ delivery of healthcare services. What has already started for emergency medicine will continue to grow in other aspects of routine delivery. In this sense, the trend is toward specializing the hospital for those procedures that have not yet reached the point where they can be delivered locally (e.g., at the site of an accident, in the home, or in an outpatient clinic). Major operations will be performed in the hospital, whereas most other delivery will be localized, low cost, and rely on technologies.

Three main transformations in information and telecommunications technologies will be crucial to achieving these trends: standardization, miniaturization, and connectivity networking. These trends will be greatly beneficial to applications in healthcare delivery, allowing for clinical (diagnostic, monitoring, and therapeutic) and administrative delivery of services in a variety of settings for a growing number of procedures and patient groups. Rural areas will benefit the most, as will pockets of the urban underprivileged.

EMERGING OR BREAKTHROUGH INNOVATIONS

The final trend is the application of emerging technologies in areas of biology, physics, and other engineering disciplines, such as mechanics and materials sciences. Never before has healthcare delivery been so open to such breakthrough technologies. Innovations in genetics and biomedical engineering, for example, are fueling a host of medical applications that are inculcated into routine delivery of services. Notwithstanding issues of ethical and moral dilemmas, American healthcare delivery, for example, is moving toward massive development of techniques, procedures, and standards in delivery of health care that is based on innovations that only a few years ago were still confined to research in laboratories. In a trend similar to that of American manufacturing during the past 20 years, in which companies have sharply reduced the time it takes to get new products from research to the market, the trend in health care is to reduce the time innovations take from the laboratory to applications in the delivery of care.

Constrained mainly by federal payors such as Medicare and Medicaid and private insurers (who usually follow in the footsteps of the government), providers are rushing innovative technologies to the bedside of their patients, in effect transforming the hospital into a "beta site" for these innovations. This trend is likely to intensify in the coming years.

In addition to the ethical issues, a key barrier to the application of emerging technologies is an acceptable definition of what constitutes "breakthrough" innovations. Difficulties in definition impact payments for procedures and services, thus requiring solutions that are agreeable to all parties to the healthcare delivery system. As emerging technologies accumulate, are tested, and are used, more such innovations enter the mainstream of medicine, leading to better and less quarrelsome ways to define breakthrough attributes of these innovations. The trend in the coming years will be to improve the system of adoption and to accelerate the acceptance of innovations for clinical usage.

Healthcare delivery is moving in the direction of becoming a technology-based activity. Whether for reasons of increased efficiency or cost savings, medical and healthcare technologies are increasingly becoming not only a pervasive presence in the sector but also a force that determines the practice of medicine and the delivery of healthcare services. Physicians and other caregivers are becoming managers, economists, and particularly technologists, albeit slowly. To deliver health care in the future will mean to be aware of the economics, the organization, and above all the technological aspects of the delivery system.

TRENDS AND DIRECTIONS IN THE HOSPITAL OF THE FUTURE

Healthcare technologies will change the architecture of hospitals, the locus of delivery of services, and the nature of the delivery process itself. It has already begun to upset the ratio of the components in the cost of delivery. As technological innovations abound in the delivery of healthcare services, the nature of clinical encounters between caregivers and patients will change, and the concepts of patient outcomes and patient value will have to be drastically redefined. A whole range of choices will be readjusted to the prevailing trends, and some are already in existence. Choices of medical procedures are, and will continue to be, influenced by cost, place of delivery (home, clinic, or hospital), and technologies applied (e.g., genetically engineered products or procedures for the diagnosis, monitoring, or cure of certain diseases and symptoms).

Although with the ubiquitous use of the Internet for healthcare applications the current wisdom suggests that patients will become more knowledgeable and empowered to make decisions about healthcare delivery, we believe that this trend will be secondary to the changes that will occur in the delivery system itself. As caregivers continue to be influenced by economics, organization, and technology, the nature of medicine will thus dramatically change, making patients' empowerment a marginal factor. Future delivery will be so dependent on the variables listed above that patients and their families will be confronted with a very limited range of possibilities, thus largely constraining their ability to be selective.

The hospital of the future may become a reality in 20 or 50 years. We believe that the concept transcends simple architectures of facilities for the delivery of care. Technology will contribute to the almost irrelevancy of the *locus* of delivery. The tremendous growth in home care and telemedicine may lead to drastic transformation of the architecture of homes to accommodate needs of healthcare delivery. These changes may include portals for technologies—creation of space for monitoring and diagnostic instrumentation, and high powered devices that today are the sole property of hospitals.

Changes are also occurring in hospice and palliative care. In the United States over 80 percent of terminal patients die in the hospital. These numbers are dropping as hospice services become more available and patients declare their desire to spend the remainder of their days at home. With the transformation in home care, there will be unparalleled growth in the home as the locus for palliative care.

The hospital of the future may also be a diversified operation, consisting of a central unit for most radical procedures, linked to a network of local "mini-hospitals." As the legal, ethical, and technical issues of distance medicine are resolved, standards of quality will be established across regions, states, and continents. Hospitals will be transformed into centers of medical knowledge and specialized skills, whereas routine medicine will be practiced in peripheral architectures and in the home.

The diversity of contributions to this book clearly illustrates the breadth of the concept of the hospital of the future. It reflects the convergence of the clinical, administrative, and hospitality dimensions of healthcare delivery. These, in turn, are mitigated by cultural, sociological, and economic attributes of communities and people.

In all of the advanced countries healthcare delivery continues to be a top priority of the political and human agenda. We are now accustomed to continuous improvements in health care, improved technologies of diagnosis and therapeutics, and the immense effort to extend life and to bring about cures for a host of diseases. Within this context, the hospital of the future will be an architecture that makes these wishes a reality—limited by economics, technological achievements, and cultural barriers.

Part I

Creating Frameworks

Chapter 1

A Network Approach to Healthcare Quality Improvement: The Case of a Finnish Hospital District

Uija Lämsä and Taina Savolainen

INTRODUCTION

In the last 20 years, interest in networking has increased rapidly as the movement toward quality has spread globally [1]. Different network theories and several approaches have been identified in the literature, such as the interorganization and actor-network theories, and policy and industrial network approaches. Although the field of these different schools of network thought is far from homogeneous and coherent, the emphasis, for the most part, has been on different exchange relationships. In the research field, actors and bonds have mostly been studied in organizations operating in the business environment.

This chapter looks at customer orientation as a significant driving force, as a "push" toward a networking way of action. As the quality movement spread throughout the public sector after the mid-1990s, the emphasis on quality improvement and total quality thinking became requirements of the network.

This chapter proposes that different competencies and capabilities develop in networks where quality is highlighted. The competence networks can be identified on three different levels/dimensions: individual, organizational, and the whole system or the entire network of intra- and interorganizational activities and processes. For example, doctors, nurses, and other employees of an organization form the organization's core competence on an individual level. Different units are part of their own organizational network structure even as they link together to form an overall network structure. All of these individual, intra-, and interorganizational elements, as well as organizational infrastructure and outside cooperative partners, are integrated in one entity of total competence. More patient-focused nursing has occurred through customer orientation as the driver for building different dimensional/multilevel networks.

This chapter identifies the concept of, and approaches to, networks and the nature and characteristics of networks in the nonprofit sector and the complex healthcare organization. Next, the meaning and importance of customer orientation is analyzed by considering what is meant by being customer led. Three real life examples are presented in the empirical section. They represent different types of suborganizations (units) in a hospital district. These cases describe the various challenges and advantages that are gained from networking.

CONCEPT OF NETWORK AND NETWORK APPROACHES

Axelsson and Easton [2] described the network as a model or metaphor that describes a number, usually a large number, of entities that are connected. In the case of social, communication, or electrical networks, the entities are actors involved in the economic processes that convert resources to finished goods and services for consumption by end users, whether they are individuals or organizations.

Networks have been approached and theoretized in many different ways in the literature. These network approaches come from various disciplines or subdisciplines: sociology, innovation studies, political science, industrial marketing and purchasing, and comparative studies of economic systems. For example, Araujo and Easton identified 10 different network approaches [3]. Although the field of different schools of network thought is far from homogeneous and coherent, the emphasis has been on different exchange relationships.

THE NATURE OF NETWORKS IN THE NONPROFIT SECTOR

Networks have mainly been studied in the coalition of organizations that operate in the business environment, with emphasis on industrial networks. For example, the well-known researcher of industrial networks, Geoffrey Easton [4], pictured industrial networks through four metaphors: networks as relationships, structures, positions, and processes. Although his focus was to examine industrial networks that are mainly profit oriented, these thoughts can be aptly applied to the more institutional and normative nonprofit network that is the focus of this research.

A network may be seen as aggregations of relationships. Relationships between organizations and units, and even between individuals in a nonprofit network, must be considered as important in determining network properties, and knowledge of their behavior has important implications for understanding networks. Relationships may be presented as comprising four elements: mutual orientation, mutual objectives, mutual bonds, and mutual investment. Mutual orientation (dependence, investments) implies that the organizations are prepared to interact with each other and will expect each other to do so [5]. The organizations operating in the nonprofit sector must have mutual objectives and missions; they must have a preparedness to interact, mutual knowledge, and respect for each other's interests. Relationships also comprise the dependence that each has, or believes it has, upon the other. The third element is the bond that exists between organizations and/or units. Bonds can be of various kinds and strengths. In network terms, strong bonds provide a more stable and predictable structure—one that is more likely to withstand change. In the nonprofit network, bonds are mostly normative, communicative, and stable, but not static. Johanson and Mattsson identified the fourth element of relationships—the investment: "Investments are processes in which resources are committed in order to create, build or acquire assets which can be used in the future" [6]. In the nonprofit network, resources, by nature, are "soft" rather than "hard"—that is, they contain more human assets (people and their relations and competencies) than traditional investments (machines) [7]. According to Lämsä [8], besides this so-called "soft" data (or resources), which is stored in people's capabilities, investments can also be traced from both internal and external social coalitions or clusters in the organization— for example, teams, groups, communities, and networks. In health care, human assets are key.

If the organizations within the network are interdependent rather than independent, then the network will have structure. The structure of nonprofit networks can be very loose so that organizations are relatively independent, with their own structures and objectives. On the other hand, they can also be strictly structured because of these organizations' mutual orientation, which could be, for example, improving and developing health care. In this kind of tightly structured network, organizations have strong bonds and clearly demarcated activities.

Networks may also be considered in the perspective of an aggregation of interlocking positions. Mattsson [9] defines a position as a role "that the organization has for other organizations that it is related to, directly or indirectly." Positions may be defined at different level of analysis— micro- and macropositions. The microposition is characterized by (1) the role of the firm in relation to the other firm(s), (2) its importance to the other firm, and (3) the strength of the relationship with the other firm. The macroposition is characterized by (1) the identity of the other firms with which the firm has direct and indirect relationships in the network,

Figure 1.1
Beyond Customer-Led Orientation

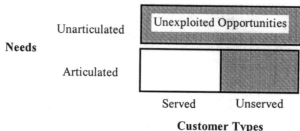

Customer Types

(2) the role of the firm in the network, and (3) the strength of the relationships with the other firms [6]. Especially in the nonprofit network, the positions between organizations or units can be very strong and strict—some organizations or units may have a very superior position in relation to the others.

Finally, networks can be seen as processes. Two dialectical processes in networks are competition and cooperation. The picture of network relationships emphasizes cooperation, complementarity, and coordination. In the nonprofit network, cooperation between various organizations often plays a significant role in their activities; the existence of strong bonding demonstrates a high level of cooperation. On the other hand, although organizations in the same network have the same mission, they often have divergent short-term objectives that create competition, for example, for various resources (like labor, equipment, or customers). In single relationships, nets and networks have to decide the trade-off between cooperation—necessary in order to create benefit—and competition over the control, ownership, or share of the resource(s) so created.

THE MEANING OF CUSTOMER ORIENTATION

There are many issues and dangers from being customer led. Hamel and Prahalad [10] claim that "customers are notoriously lacking in foresight." But recent developments in the world have changed customer perceptions so that people are more aware of what is happening in the development of organizations [11]. The same is true for the healthcare sector customers (local health centers as well as individual patients). Customers have become more aware of quality care and are more capable of articulating their hopes and needs. Hamel and Prahalad [10] present a simple two-by-two matrix (see Figure 1.1) where one axis represents needs—those that customers are capable of articulating and those that they can't yet articulate. The other axis represents classes of customer—

those classes that the organization currently serves and those that it does not. However well an organization meets the articulated needs of current customers, it runs a great risk if it doesn't have a view of the needs customers can't yet articulate, but would love to have satisfied.

But why is it worth paying attention to the importance of customers? What advantages and benefits can be gained from listening to the customers' point of view? Next we present three real life examples that show the kinds of challenges and problems these organizations faced when building their networks and the opportunities and benefits they gained from networking. Customer orientation, especially, has worked as a significant driving force, as a "push" toward a networking way of action. Also, the importance of quality and integrated quality thinking (total quality) clearly becomes important when building the competence network.

THE CASE OF A FINNISH HOSPITAL DISTRICT

Northern Ostrobothnia Hospital District (PPSHP) is a coalition of organizations that "produces" special medical treatment in the region of Oulu. Besides caring for patients, the capabilities and core competencies include teaching and research work, material services, and the emergency duties of 22 local communities. The PPSHP operates three hospitals: Oulu University Hospital, Oulaskangas Hospital, and Visala Hospital. It also is responsible for the communal organization of health centers (basic public health services) under national health law. The basic idea is that the local communities will buy the services of special medical treatment from PPSHP so that customers come into the hospitals by referrals from health centers. Besides patients, the customers of PPSHP are local communities, health centers, other units of social and public health services, and also the educational establishments, such as the University of Oulu. Nowadays, the PPSHP has defined the patient as the most important customer, even if the local community pays for the services. In the past, this perspective was different: patients were merely one of many customers.

The development of quality has been divided into different spheres of responsibility. The top hierarchy consists of the Director and Council of the Hospital District. Next is the Chief Surgeon (the manager of quality management) who is in charge of quality development. The next layer contains the quality coordinator who plans and organizes the implementation of the whole development of quality. In each profit center, organizations have their own quality manager and, in each sphere of responsibilities, a position in charge of quality. People in charge of quality are key in the quality development and continuously communicate

Figure 1.2
The Competence Networks

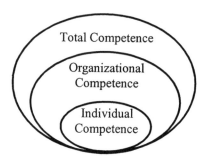

with each other as the objective is to develop and improve the transfer of knowledge and know-how—to learn from others.

Figure 1.2 demonstrates the three different levels/dimensions of the competence networks: individual, organizational-unit, and the whole system of intra- and interorganizational activities and processes. Doctors, nurses, and other employees of the organization form the organization's core competence on the individual level. For a long time, doctors have had their own intranet where they shared experiences, information, and research results. The several units of PPSHP are part of their own organizational network structure and, at the same time, form an overall network structure. The external cooperation partners and interest groups are, for example, pharmaceutical industries, material services, research centers, and infrastructure services. All individuals, intra- and interorganizational elements with organizations' infrastructure and outside cooperative partners are integrated in one entity of total competence. Customer orientation as a driver for building different dimensional/multilevel networks has led to more patient-focused nursing. The more intensive cooperation between individuals and units has improved the organization's core process of care (e.g., the planning of care, following the progress of the patient) and has led to increased feedback from patients. The developing network with its more effective activities has improved the organization of follow-up care for patients.

Oulu University Hospital

Oulu University Hospital is the northernmost of five university central hospitals in Finland. The hospital currently provides treatment for the people in the Northern Ostrobothnia Hospital District and Northern Finland in general. It also offers international services to Scandinavia and other parts of the world. The hospital cooperates closely with the adjacent Medipolis center, a concentration of medical and biotechnical companies, and the Kastelli Research Center. Other units on the same premises are the WHO Collaborating Center for Research in Human Reproduction and the Population and Family Welfare Federation's Fertility Clinic. However, the hospital's special emphasis is on personal treatment for each patient.

In Oulu University Hospital, some level of internal networking between different units and departments has traditionally existed. However, networking has not been very tight and has played a minor role in practice. In the past, patients were treated in one unit, but consulting work was received from other units with written consulting application when needed. But the total quality thinking has changed this, and care is now more patient oriented. Especially when talking about the patient who requires the treatment of several different sectors, there is a need for tight but flexible collaboration between these sectors. Also, the planning and gradation of care has brought some smoothness into operations, which means that patients are in the right place at the right time, and they don't have to stay in Oulu University Hospital too long because further care is arranged within the patient's own local area.

The Psychiatry Clinic

The Psychiatry Clinic is part of Oulu University Hospital, and it has a lot of cooperation (e.g., exchange of information and different cooperative projects) with Visala Hospital because of their common concentration on psychiatry. Several health centers, local communities, and the provincial administrative board are also members of the network of the Psychiatry Clinic and have established essential cooperative relationships with each other. The provincial administrative board has a unique role in this network: its duty is to coordinate and organize different cooperative projects and conduct control visits to the units and departments of the Hospital District. The Psychiatry Clinic is a public organization that operates under the nation's laws, regulations, orders, book of instructions, and so forth. This unit produces knowledge and know-how, and uses this intellectual capital in its services.

Because of the huge amount of norms and standards, the development and operation of this unit is much more restricted in comparison with common business organizations. Also, the structure of this unit, which is very hierarchical and contains different types of organization models, sets constraints on development. A specific problem has been the combination of hierarchical, expert, and process organization, mainly because there is confusion and lack of clarity about how the responsibilities are allocated at different times according to the organizational model. The unit has nearly completed the ISO 9001 quality system implementation, and this action has brought considerable benefits. For example, the quality of documentation has improved, and concrete control of many unit norms have been established. Although the structure of this unit has been criticized, this multiform and divided structure also has been seen as being very beneficial. For example, the research and development unit gives expert guidance to the Psychiatry Clinic by helping it to improve its quality of care. One objective is to produce good quality scientific research while also improving the quality of clinical work. It is noteworthy that quality is also being developed through customer feedback, which is received through inquiry forms, telephone calls, and e-mail. It is crucial that personnel regard quality as important and as the factor that clarifies their operations.

Eye Clinic

The Eye Clinic also operates as a part of Oulu University Hospital. The objective of this unit is to compact the collaboration between independent profit centers, making it more intensive and reducing overlapping work. Besides health centers and local communities (legally required to be members), other eye clinics, (e.g., the clinics of Kemi and Kajaani) are also members of the Eye Clinic's network. This cooperation, however, is not very systematic nor advanced. Internally, the clinic has networked quite well because it has developed its activities into self-directed teams. These teams are not totally independent but get their tasks from the organization's upper levels. Although teams are able to develop the operations of the clinic, the budget responsibility remains in the profit center. For years, the special focus has been in the development of quality. The clinic conducts self-assessments based on the criteria of the Finnish Quality Award, identifying both its strengths and the areas for improvement. Customer feedback and various other inquiries play a significant part in the clinic's development.

The development of quality has also faced some problems in the Eye Clinic. First of all, personnel often have difficulty understanding that customer quality should be as extensive as purely technical quality. Furthermore, the development of quality takes time from other functions, and it has been frequently discovered that "quality language"—where open discussion and listening to criticism are important to further quality development—doesn't seem to suit the hospital environment

SUMMARY AND CONCLUSION

Is it possible to see the customer as first in the hospital of the future? And are there advantages to be gained from networking? The answer could be yes, but the organization must have strong know-how, strong core competencies, and developed capabilities. The relationship with the customer should be multiform and trustful. Both parties should have at least a certain level of commitment in the relationships. In order for medical care to work fluently from the customer's point of view, there is a need for more intensive cooperation between different units. The importance of personnel is seen as one of the most essential components in developing quality; if the personnel are not committed to mutual objectives, the system cannot work. The attitude of cooperation partners has been appreciative and, particularly, the meaning of transferring of knowledge and communication has been realized. The most critical problems in developing quality and building a network are the lack of resources (mostly time), attitudes and prejudices, and the conflicts between basic public health and special medical treatment, mainly in allocation of activities.

The idea of a real network and its development was introduced over a decade ago. However, only in recent years has the development of a network become one of the keystone objectives for the Northern Ostrobothnia Hospital District. Quality thinking, quality development, and a more advanced customer-oriented operation can be seen as fundamental principles for building a network in the organization. A team for continuous quality improvement has also been organized to build a quality system for the use of the whole coalition of organizations. The first actions have already been undertaken. The objectives of the personnel training is to teach process thinking to employees, especially looking at processes from the patient's perspective.

NOTES

[1] Savolainen, T., "Development of Quality-Oriented Management Ideology: A Longitudinal Case Study on the Permeation of Quality Ideology in Two Finnish Family-Owned Manufacturing Companies," *Economics and Statistics* (Jyväskylä, Finland: University of Jyväskylä, 1997).

[2] Axelsson, B., and G. Easton (Eds.), *Industrial Networks: A New View of Reality* (London: Routledge, 1992).

[3] Araujo, J., and G. Easton, "Networks in Socioeconomic Systems: A Critical Review," in Iacobucci, D. (Ed.), *Networks in Marketing* (Thousand Oaks, CA: Sage Publications, 1996), pp. 63–107.

[4] Easton, G., "Industrial Networks: A Review," in Axelsson, B., and G. Easton (Eds.), *Industrial Networks: A New View of Reality* (London: Routledge, 1992), pp. 3–27.

[5] Mattsson, L., "Interaction Strategies: A Network Approach," AMA Marketing Educator's Conference, San Francisco, CA, 1988.

[6] A. Johanson and L. Mattsson, "Interorganizational Relations in Industrial Systems: A Network Approach Compared with a Transaction Cost Approach," University of Uppsala, Sweden, 1986.

[7] Savolainen, T., "Towards a New Workplace Culture: Development Strate-

gies for Employer-Employee Relations," *The Journal of Workplace Learning*, 12(8), 2000, 318–326.

[8] Lämsä, U., "Using Knowledge Management in Improving the Quality of the Development Processes," Conference Proceedings of the Fourth International Software & Internet Quality 2000, Software Research Institute, San Francisco, CA, November 20–24, 2000.

[9] Mattsson, L., "An Application of a Network Approach to Marketing: Defending and Changing Market Positions," in Dholakia, N., and J. Arndt (Eds.), *Changing the Course of Marketing: Alternative Paradigms for Widening Marketing Theory* (Greenwich, CT: JAI Press, 1984).

[10] Hamel, G., and C. Prahalad, *Competing for the Future* (Boston: The Harvard Business School Press, 1994).

[11] Lämsä, U., "Towards a Learning Organization—Understanding the Factors That Influence Progress," Case Organization Fortum Service Ltd., Faculty of Economics and Industrial Management, Oulu University, Oulu, Finland, 2000.

Chapter 2

The Industrial Product versus the Facility Product: A Framework for Crystallizing the Healthcare Services of Tomorrow

Jan-Erik Gasslander, Tomas Engström, and Åke Wiklund

BACKGROUND

The building design (and construction) process (comprising the planning, building, and maintenance phases) of healthcare facilities is a complex process. Traditionally, the practices and logic employed by the building trade regulate this process with questionable results. One approach that could be used to help avoid the sometimes unfortunate results of such a traditional process is to take advantage of experiences from other branches of industry. However, in order to be successful, this method demands a way of generalizing that will retain the specific details and characteristics of those different branches. This calls for linking the discourse to the ongoing design paradigm and design criteria within the branches involved.

The restructuring of the healthcare sector to bring it in line with technical development is also dictated by lack of appropriate personnel resources. This fact will in the future further underline the need for a nontraditional way of organizing the building design process. This will, in turn, affect the services provided by the so-called core business within the healthcare sector, which is mainly carried out by doctors and nurses. The patients' insights regarding medical matters are gradually improving. At the same time, various achievements are taking place in the field of science, such as an accelerating development of computer-based expert systems supported by various distance communications systems (e.g., telemedicine). The patient's role will be transformed in future with patients contributing to a greater extent to the services provided (this process of change might humorously be termed "seeing your doctor by remote control").

To keep up with this accelerating process of change, new approaches to supplying appropriate building facilities for the core business are needed. This will obviously, in turn, affect various existing and new auxiliary support functions, leading to totally new organizational and technical interfaces being defined.

It is the aim of this chapter to contribute to this process of change by utilizing other sectors as a comparison, namely, the automotive industry, which might function as a catalyst. This comparison will involve the traditional building design process as such, as well as give an outline of some characteristics of the "facility product" of the future, as applied to the healthcare sector. All this is in many respects a process change that has already been started in Sweden.

The authors' recent experiences concerning participation in the building design processes of university buildings underline the need to transform the traditional building facility (the "facility product") by means of established industrial product development methods into a more advanced product. It will thereby be possible to define yet another product for analytical purposes, namely the "industrial product."

The healthcare sector in Sweden is also affected by anomalies in which user (tenant) participation during building design has encountered extensive resistance (see [1] and [2]). In none of the cases reported in these studies was the researcher able to identify any example in which the responsible official decision makers had reformed their formal decision procedure in accordance with the healthcare personnel's time schedule [2]. To summarize, in Sweden substantial resources have been invested in various forms of participative initiatives within the healthcare sector. Unfortunately, however, these initiatives have not proved especially constructive.

The newly popularized term of facilities management [3], which is a reorientation of the building trade (and thereby the healthcare building facilities), may, or may not, be used to denote this transformation of the "facility product" that has become more or less a necessity due to circumstances dealt with below.

AIMS AND DELIMITATIONS

This chapter focuses on generalization by discussing the "facility product" and the "industrial product" in their respective professional contexts. In this respect it should be noted that the Swedish government has recently approved the term "value chain" as a constructive concept for the recent development within industry. This development was hardly something that the building trade had anticipated [4]. Thus, the exploration of the "facility product" by means of industrial references is only in its infancy, even though there are a few examples (see, e.g., [5] and [6]).

On the other hand, experiences from industry, especially those from various product development processes, shape a different practice and logic. There, the process of, for example, defining and integrating user (customer) demands in the process, where resources and costs are carefully monitored, has, according to some of the authors' experiences, in most respects, no correspondence within the building trade [7]. It may be argued that the industrial mass production process is not applicable to the design of customized products such as buildings. This statement might to some extent be true. However, the mirroring of the practices and logic of other sectors is likely to elucidate potentials as well as discrepancies in a way that would otherwise be unexplored.

Thus, the authors will compare the two sectors mentioned above at both the general and specific levels. This, in combination with the restructuring of the healthcare sector briefly touched upon above, implies a new infrastructure of various healthcare facilities that particularly exploit telemedicine and information technology.

INDUSTRIAL FRAMES OF REFERENCE

The frames of reference referred to in this chapter concern industrial product development and, to some extent, also assembly system design. These frames of reference could, in the local research context of the authors, be seen as amalgamating various aspects of manufacturing in order to link the production system design to the building facility. Such an approach has been treated by Granath [8], who has studied the linkage between production system design and building facility design for a selected number of cases.

However, the most spectacular and far-reaching industrial restructuring referred to in this chapter concerns the use of a specific design procedure that has been refined and used by some of the authors in five cases within the automotive industry. This work involved long-term cooperation between industry and university [7]. In most of these cases it has been a matter of design of unorthodox assembly systems. These assembly systems comprised parallel product flow, long cycle time assembly systems, which are the opposites of serial product flow, and short cycle time assembly systems (i.e., the traditional assembly line) [9]. These insights are scientifically proven and empirically validated but not yet fully established internationally [10].

On the other hand, the frames of reference regarding industrial product development processes represent knowledge that is well established within international industry (see, for example, [11] or [12]). However, these need to be complemented with one of the authors' professional experiences concerning industrial product development of professional products (articulated vehicles and sawmills). These insights comprise methods for the procedure to pass a product through the phases of product development, production, purchasing, and marketing [11], [13], [14]. Focus groups indicate a further recognition of user (customer) demands having an influence on industrial product development processes (user controlled product development). Such groups have, for instance, been used for developing vehicles for public transportation, including vehicles for distribution of goods within a city [15].

In short, the product development process within the industry comprises allocation of defined functions to the physical product, which in turn will create functions recognized by the user (customer). This means that, in order to be fulfilled, functions and services have to be specified and some of them allocated to services provided by professional personnel. In some cases, a product might consist, mainly or solely, of provided services. In this case it might be suitable to talk about a "service product" [16].

CHARACTERIZING THE "FACILITY PRODUCT" OF TODAY

Applying the introduced industrial frames of reference to the building facility makes it possible to recognize the "facility product." In a narrow sense, this may be interpreted as allocating defined functions to be fulfilled by selected building functions that are created by the building facility.

However, apart from supplying the appropriate building facilities for the core business, it is, in a broader sense, necessary to recognize the need for various forms of support functions for the "facility product," along the lines of the practice already established within the industry. As mentioned above, this fact calls for the definition of new organizational and technical interfaces.

Generally speaking, for the user (tenant) of the building facility, the definition of the product as such in the form of the physical building has for a long time been unclear. This situation is, according to some of the authors' experiences, a distinctive feature of university buildings. This situation is basically due to a deficient dialogue between user (tenant), the persons responsible for the specific building design, and the university's property manager. All these idiosyncrasies emanate from the property owner (i.e., the university), whose qualifications as a customer, responsible for defining the building facilities, have proved to be poor. Nevertheless, the resulting building costs are perplexing (see [17]). Verification processes comprising user (tenant) participation are, according

Figure 2.1
Some Comparisons between the "Industrial Product" and the "Facility Product"

	The "Industrial Product"	The "Facility Product" of Today
Market Characteristics	• Market research is mostly carried out. • For consumer products strong competition exists. • For professional products and complete production systems there is an oligopoly situation.	• Delimited market research is carried out. • An oligopolistic situation or most often a monopolistic situation.
Product Development Characteristics	• Fast product development for consumer products. • Slower product development for professional products and commodities.	• Slow product development since driving forces are mostly lacking. • Rational and systematic methods for product development exist but are mostly not used.
Product Verification Characteristics	• Very complex and time-consuming product verifications, which are generally carried out. • The user (customer) takes part directly in the verification process, even in the early phases.	• Verification processes comprising user (tenant) participation is rare. • The user (tenant) does not always take part in the early phases.*

*The critical function of a correctly designed and utilized building program, as an integrated part of the more traditional building design documentation, must be emphasized. This program must be constructed and communicated in the early phases of the building design process and has to be recognized by all persons involved (see, e.g., [18]).

to some of the authors' experiences, rare. Generally speaking, the design of public buildings in Sweden is hampered by shortcomings. This especially concerns the dialogue between persons responsible for investments in building facilities [19].

Figure 2.1 illuminates the intriguing problem area of defining various key terms in both the long- and short-term perspective, respectively. For example, the customer of an automobile will consider, among other things, the trade-in value of the vehicle. On the other hand, the user (tenant) of the "facility product" must consider the future reformation of his or her activities in a somewhat shorter perspective than the property owner. The comparison between the two "products" above also underlines the difference in time perspective between the two branches involved. The product development phase of vehicles comprises, for example, three to six years, after which it may be marketed at a profit for a period of 5 to 10 years. The building design process represents a marginal part of the building facilities' "profitable life."

This fact could be exemplified as follows: a customer seeks a product that satisfies his or her demands. The building facility of tomorrow (including various associated installations) therefore needs, to a larger degree than today, to be modified to meet even more shifting demands due to changing activities of the user (tenant) and other circumstances not dictated by the user (tenant), such as various political processes (i.e., changing "political contracts"). This implies possibilities to increase the profit generated by the "facility product" as well as for the core business of the user (tenant), since the user (tenant) only demands to purchase specific support functions needed during a specific period of time.

Thus, the building trade of the future will most certainly be transformed from a monopolistic to a more oligopolistic situation. The future development of the "facility product" will thus have much in common with industrial product development processes. However, since the "facility product" also contains extensive elements of service supplied to professional users (tenants), an accelerating development of the service dimensions will take place. This accelerating development will specifically be applicable in cases where the professional user (tenant) is prepared to invest his own resources in the early phases of the building design process. This insight has, according to some of the authors' experiences, not been prominent during the design of university buildings.

According to one of the authors' experiences regarding assembly system design, the most far-sighted developers of the "facility product" must recognize the need to refine their knowledge by using various forms of documentation beyond the traditional design documentation.

This type of product specification of the building facility is far reaching, stretching from the start of the building design to the user (tenant) occupying the building. It corresponds to automotive product specifications in the form of product data included in a product structure (see Chapter 14).

EMERGENCE OF THE "FACILITY PRODUCT" OF THE FUTURE AS APPLIED TO THE HEALTHCARE SECTOR

There are obvious similarities between the industrial product development process and the development of new healthcare services. They both contain concentrated activities during a given time with a given set of objectives, where a number of persons with expert competencies in a structured way develop a product with a given methodology.

Professional personnel responsible for developing the "industrial product" have a role that is similar to their counterparts in charge of healthcare service development. This is especially evident when the industrial product development process comprises so-called user-friendly products. Note also that it is in fact a layman who is the consumer of the healthcare services, which is also true for the "industrial product" in the case of consumer products.

In the authors' opinion, one of the merits of applying established industrial product development methods within the healthcare sector, such as focus groups, is that this will probably legitimize the restructuring briefly discussed in the first section. A similar analysis for the healthcare service of the future, in accordance with the "service product," is also possible. Here, of course, certain unique characteristics have to be considered, such as privacy, personal integrity, ethical circumstances, and so forth [20, 21].

To summarize, the healthcare sector of the future has to restructure. The work to accomplish this may, or may not, utilize industrial frames of reference. If these references are put to use, they will probably legitimize the restructuring, as will, of course, various achievements in the field of science. However, this process of change will, most certainly, also contribute to a much more inclusive definition of the healthcare services. It should be noted that some of the ideas and concepts brought forward in this chapter are by no means new. For example, the healthcare service that is specifically aimed at the patients is described by Graf [22], who focuses on reduced queues, while Petersson [23] concentrates on "the patient in focus."

CONCLUSIONS AND FINAL COMMENT

This chapter has specifically discussed the building design process in general, using the terms the "industrial product" and the "facility product" (see Figure 2.1). By taking advantage of general design criteria, it proved possible to crystallize some characteristics of the "facility product" of the future, as applied to the healthcare sector (see Figure 2.2).

Figure 2.2 explains the internal communication and relationships (codified as [A] in the figure) in combination with the external communication and relationships with the organization surrounding the product (codified as [B] in the figure). An organization that provides products and/or services to various users (customers) is based on a product design process that is a result of a more or less formalized process (codified as [C] in the figure). The application of these design criteria results in a more efficient product (codified as [D] in the figure).

As is evident in Figure 2.2, the industrial frames of reference should be transferable to the "facility product." This transfer must, however, recognize that the time perspective of the building trade is shorter than

Figure 2.2
Industrial Frames of Reference

Specification of general design criteria appropriate for both industry and the healthcare sector. These criteria have been applied to healthcare building facilities in Sweden (e.g., the hospital in Karlstad).

Design Criteria to Achieve Defined Functions	Established Methods Applied for the Industrial Product of Today	Some Characteristics of the Facility Product of the Future as Applied to the Healthcare Sector
(A) Internal communication and relationships within the organization.	• Product managers—responsible for specific products/product families. • Specific education and training in marketing/manufacturing departments in accordance with product specification.	• Facility manager—responsible for total facilities/building facilities. • Facility staff training and education in accordance with corporate policies/contract specifications.
(B) External communication and relationships between the organization and user.	• Focus groups to articulate user demands, noted above. • Test marketing to measure and verify user acceptance. • Market research/estimation to measure market potential.	• Focus groups to articulate user demands comprising professional personnel.
(C) Product design process.	• Function analysis in accordance with integrated product development. • Comprehensive specification of demands; consensus of design, manufacturing, purchasing, and marketing departments, which includes user demands and environmental restrictions.	• Function analysis with so-called integrated product development. Analysis to include implications from the political process (i.e., a "political contract"). • Comprehensive specification of demands, a consensus monitoring defined interface between facility manager and user.
(D) Efficiency due to factors such as maintenance, costs, space utilization, etc., which is effect of A–C above.	• Achieved by so-called value analyses (i.e., cost versus function). • User value versus market segment.	• Value analysis in conjunction with user and marketing departments at facility supplier to define functions to include in "facility product," considering consequences in form of costs. • User value versus market segment; corresponds to hospital departments with different budgets to spend on "facility product."

within industry. The building design process (comprising the planning, building, and maintenance phases) is a matter of some years. After this time, some of the traditional building design representatives (building design participators), such as designers, main contractors, and subcontractors, leave the property owner, property managers, and user (tenant) with the completed building in order to initiate yet another building design process elsewhere.

There are, in fact, new forms of legal contracts under discussion for building facilities that are rented by professional users (tenants). These forms are chiseling out various functional aspects, such as responsibilities for various building systems and maintenance aspects. Another consideration aimed at the professional user (tenant) is to establish long-term contracts. This sometimes includes a deposit sum for specific services and functions (e.g., during a 10-year period).

Example

In large Swedish hospitals built in the 1960s and onwards, the development of expensive technical equipment, combined with a general belief in the economic advantages of "large-scale production," caused a concentration of resources for diagnostics, treatment, and service of centralized buildings. This concept relied on proximity and straightforward communication between various departments within the hospital. Large, connected structures of an unimaginable scale arose within the healthcare sector, where the patients were moved around like "goods by a distribution firm."

As a result of this development, master plans were developed for hospitals that distinguish between different zones, such as "inpatient ward" for patients staying for more than one day, "outpatient ward," and "treatment facilities." All of these zones called for defined concentrated locations of their own in the building. Therefore, separate buildings were designed with a high degree of internal flexibility. Thus, hospitals were, as a whole, given an inherited static design that was not amenable to various types of reformations. This fact is evident for many existing hospitals today.

Nevertheless, new concepts for organizing medical services that exploit the potentials of highly specialized medical services are being successively developed. At the same time, a number of more autonomous and more complete small-scale organizations focused on medical specialities like cardiology, neurology, and orthopedics are being concentrated in various types of centers [24, 25].

The internationally proclaimed idea of "patient-focused care" is another concept that gives rise to new user (tenant) demands on the building facility. Briefly explained, this concept implies that doctors, nurses, equipment, and other types of resources will come to the patients wherever they are. In the most extreme case, this means that the resources are brought to the patient. This is in contrast to the "large-scale production" of the 1960s. It is, however, also possible to identify a generic healthcare building facility, which is composed of a mixture of the large- and small-scale concepts.

To summarize, the master plan for the hospital of the future will successively be reformed into organ-based centers that have a building of their own, along the line of a campus area. The patients would only be moved around in the hospital in exceptional cases—for example, when there is a need for highly specialized diagnostic equipment or treatment. The university hospital in Trondheim, Norway, which is under design, is an actual example.

In the specific buildings for such a center, there are beds and equipment as well as possibilities for diagnostics, treatment, and rehabilitation. The building also acts as a center for follow-up care in direct contact with the patient on an out-patient basis combined with facilities for out-patient treatment and home care. It is also a center for close cooperation with the patient's own local care center and family doctor, as some urban districts are sometimes situated in another urban district.

An individual building located in an organ-based center can gain an identity of its own by means of its own entrances, which are easy for the patients to find, while its smaller scale also makes it more comprehensible to the patient. With the aid of telemedicine, digitalized radiology, and so forth, various medical specialists are able to cooperate with doctors in smaller hospitals and local care centers that are located far away.

Thus, the hospital of the future will not just be a hospital as we recognize it today; it will be a hub in a decentralized network serving patients not only in the hospital but also in local hospitals and, to a much greater extent than at present, in their homes.

This example illustrates the two different concepts of building facilities for the healthcare sector, concepts that in turn might be interpreted to reflect assembly system design in industry. The "zone-plan hospital" is a reflection of an industrial process promoting movements of the product inside the building (i.e., the assembly line requires large-scale building facilities). The "campus-plan hospital" mirrors a more up-to-date parallel product flow assembly system, comprising small, autonomous work groups completing the vehicles being manufactured. In the latter case, it is not the products' movements in the building that govern what really happens, but the intra–work group pattern of the operators, as they are the ones who contribute their services to the product. By analogy, the different medical professionals are concentrated around one patient. To conclude, it is the authors' opinion that there is a great deal to learn about design of healthcare facilities from interaction between the two sectors discussed in this chapter.

NOTES

[1] Henriksson J., B. Gardell, and A. Mächs, *Eckeröprojektet 1982–1991* (Stockholm, Sweden: Jan Henriksson Arkitektkontor AB, 1983).

[2] Gustafsson, R.-Å., A. Carlsson, and J. Henriksson, *Kan vården demokratiseras* (Stockholm, Sweden: Arbetslivscentrum, 1991).

[3] Facilities management represents the extended service that a responsible facility manager can give the users. The name has much in common with the content of the different phases within a traditional building design process that are described by Wikforss and Lundequist (*Byggforskningsrådets*, G18, 1996). See [24].

[4] SOU, "Sammanfattning och förslag, Särtryck av Byggkostnadsdelegationens Slutbetänkande," *Byggkostnadsdelegationen*, SOU 2000:44, Stockholm (in Swedish), 2000.

[5] Bergqvist, L.-G., and M. Rönn, "Att flytta—Rum för nya tankar," *Chalmers Tekniska Högskola och Ortopediska Kliniken, Regionsjukhuset i Örebro* (in Swedish), 1997.

[6] Holmberg, G., "Effektivare operationsplanering," SPRI-rapport 396, Stockholm, 1995.

[7] Engström, T., D. Jonsson, and L. Medbo (2000), "The Method of Successive Assembly System Design: Six Case Studies Within the Swedish Automotive Industry," in Gunarsekaran, A. (Ed.), *Agile Manufacturing: 21st Century Manufacturing Strategy* (New York: Elsevier Science Publishers, 2001).

[8] Granath, J. Å., "Architecture, Technology and Human Factors—Design in a Sociotechnical Context," Ph.D. Thesis, Industrial Architecture and Planning, Chalmers University of Technology, Göteborg, Sweden, 1991.

[9] The introduction of unorthodox assembly systems called for a reformed product perception by operators and engineers. This proved possible to achieve by reforming the product information, which was already available in the traditional design-oriented product structure, and complementing it with data regarding the existing product and the manufacturing process to create an assembly-oriented product structure. This reformation is an essential requirement, since it facilitates the design procedure and promotes the introduction of nontraditional materials feeding techniques (i.e., it is necessary for the function of the new assembly system to communicate with the traditional design-oriented product structure). See [10] and [7].

[10] Medbo, L., "Materials Supply and Product Descriptions for Assembly System—Design and Operation," Ph.D. Thesis, Department of Transportation and Logistics, Chalmers University of Technology, Göteburg, Sweden, 1999.

[11] Olsson, F., "Systematisk Konstruktion," Ph.D. Thesis, Institutionen för Maskinkonstruktion, Lunds Tekniska Högskola, 1976.

[12] Pugh, S., *Total Design: Integrated Methods for Successful Product Engineering* (Reading, MA: Addison-Wesley, 1990).

[13] Andreasen, M., and L. Hein, *Integrated Product Development* (New York: Springer Verlag, 1987).

[14] Ulrich, K. T., and S. D. Eppinger, *Product Design and Development* (New York: Irwin/McGraw-Hill, 2000).

[15] Warsen, L., "Planering av låggolvsbussar, pendeltåg T-banetåg," *Transportforskningskommissionen (TFK)*, TFK-rapport 1996:2 (in Swedish), 1996.

[16] Grönroos, C., "Relationship Marketing: Interaction Dialogue and Value," *Svenska Handelshögskolan*, Helsingfors, 1997.

[17] Lundholm, A.-M., "Kris hotar Naturhistoriska Riksmuseet. 40 medarbetare kan få sluta. Regeringen kompenserar inte inflationen. Hyran tar halva anslaget," *Svenska Daglandet*, 11 Juni 1996, p. 15.

[18] Steen, J., and P. Ullmark, *En egen väg—Att göra fackliga arbetsmiljöprogram* (Stockholm: Kungliga Tekniska Högskolan, doktorsavhandling, 1982.

[19] Oresten, B., and K. Löfvenberg, *Rätt beslut. Investeringsbeslut i offentliga organisationer* (Stockholm: Svenska Kommunförbundet, 1998).

[20] Eriksson, K., *Vårdandets ide* (Stockholm: Almqvist & Wiksell, 1987).

[21] Eriksson, K., *Vårdprocessen* (Stockholm: Norstedts Förlag, 1988).

[22] Graf, W., "Köfri sjukvård en framtidsvision?" *Närkes Allehanda*, 12 Juni 1965.

[23] Petersson, K., "Framtidens sjukhus. Har människan mer i centrum," *Expressen*, 21 Februari 1964 p. 14.

[24] Wikforss, Ö., and J. Lundequist, "Planerings-, bygg-och förvaltningsprocessen. Byggforskningsrådets program-och uppföljningsgrupp för planerings-, bygg-och förvaltningsprocessen," *Byggforskningsrådet*, 1996, p. G18.

[25] Wiklund, Å., *Vårdens och vårdens byggnader i ständig förändring* (Stockholm: Arkitekturforskning, 2002).

Chapter 3

Mobilizing Expectations on EPR: The Case of Spain

Cecilia Cabello and Luis Sanz-Menendez

INTRODUCTION

The development of the electronic patient record (EPR) in Europe has caused extensive debate. Many policy documents and studies have addressed the various technical, social, and legal factors involved in the development and adoption of EPR for national healthcare services [1]. The approach of this chapter is to analyze the specific social-technical context of Spain, showing how the relationship and interactions among the various stakeholders, promoted through a professional organization, have successfully mobilized expectations on EPR [2].

We studied the development of health informatics in Spain, taking into consideration the interactions between three independent but overlapping systems: the healthcare system, the industrial system, and the research and technological development system. The purpose was to construct a social-technical configuration of actors involved in the development of health informatics in Spain to understand the context in which research, development, and innovation activities were carried out as a result of their relationships and interactions. In addition, we analyzed a series of factors within the configuration, including future expectations of the development of this technological sector, perceived problems or obstacles to achieve future developments, and resource dependencies or needs for research, development, and innovation activities.

To achieve these objectives, we first identified a series of key actors, including firms, public healthcare officials, public/academic researchers, and healthcare professionals. Second, we carried out in-depth interviews to study the factors mentioned above.

In the first part of this chapter we briefly discuss the background in the development of health informatics in the Spanish healthcare system, focusing primarily on INSALUD, which is the main national healthcare provider [3]. The second part of the chapter presents the results of our fieldwork, where we have constructed the social-technical network that centers around the Spanish health informatics sector, discussing the main findings with respect to the expectations, obstacles, and needs related to the future development of information technologies in health care. The final section reflects on how future expectations, mediated through the main professional organization, have mobilized actors toward adoption and diffusion of health informatics technology, primarily related to EPR.

DEVELOPMENT OF HEALTH INFORMATICS IN SPAIN

The modernization process for the Spanish healthcare system began in the late 1980s and continued in the 1990s with a government initiative called Dotación de Informática para Areas Sanitaria, or DIAS Project (provision of informatics for healthcare areas). This is when the government promoted the use of information technology systems within the healthcare service and is the moment that captures the origin of health informatics for Spanish hospitals. Exceptions occurred because some departments in a few hospitals had isolated computerized systems. The project was executed in the territory of INSALUD, the main healthcare service, which then covered most of the Spanish regions (it included 13 regions of the 17 total, but now some competencies in healthcare have been transferred) [4].

The initiative to modernize health care by implementing hospital information systems did not merely consist of purchasing or installing new technology but implied organizational changes and the setting of technological standards. The DIAS initiative involved organizational innovation and cultural changes, and can be considered an inflection point in the development of health informatics in Spain.

The outcomes following the four-year initiative of the DIAS Project are subject to some controversy. For many of those involved, it was a positive experience that set standards for Spanish hospitals in terms of technology and organization. In addition, it also changed the mentality of many doctors and hospital administrators in terms of how patient care can be more effectively achieved through the use of informatics.

However, for others, it was a negative experience because the implementation process was undertaken improperly and resulted in many unexpected problems. Some hospitals were not prepared for the changes and did not have the qualified personnel to adopt the new technologies or use them correctly and successfully. In addition, there was no follow-up effort to continue what was started. Many firms, therefore, have continued their business by simply maintaining or renewing systems.

In the last decade in Spain, the application of information and communication technologies in the health sector have evolved, as in other countries, from hospital information systems geared primarily for administrative and management purposes to those applications that have more clinical and diagnostic uses. Many hospitals have information systems that handle tasks such as admission, discharge, payroll, catering, appointments, and other administrative or management-related aspects. Analytical data and diagnostic tools (radiology, ultrasound, etc.) are more recent technological adoptions. In general, the focus has shifted to modernization processes for informatics systems in Spanish hospitals, while primary care has until recently remained relatively ignored.

In Spain, the development of health informatics in primary care contrasts somewhat with its development in other countries. For example, in the United Kingdom and the Netherlands, general practitioners in primary care (GPs) have implemented informatics systems and have electronically stored data for their patients [5]. Most GPs in these countries use computers on a regular basis, while this is not the case in Spain. This can be attributed in some part to the fact that GPs in some other countries are more autonomous, having some financial and economic independence in implementing new technologies, while in Spain the decision-making structure and resources of GPs depend entirely on the healthcare service.

The importance of healthcare informatics has been reflected by the evolution in public expenditures, which have been quite significant. During the four-year period 1993–1996, the total expenditures were only 30 million euro, however, the budget for 1997–2000 reached over 200 million euro. This budget corresponds to several initiatives, which have the following overall objectives: to improve patient care and quality, to increase the efficiency of the health care centers (both primary and specialized) by providing technology for management improvement, and to obtain aggregated information that may help to improve the services provided by the INSALUD.

This increase in expenditures and interest has promoted integration of information technology systems within hospitals. As a consequence of this evolution, decision-making mechanisms for the use and implementation of health informatics in Spain have also changed. Initially, it was the various hospital services or departments that made decisions on what informatics technologies were needed; later it was the hospital directors. Currently, most decisions are made at the centralized level—that is, by the various regional healthcare services. The various healthcare services in Spain have set up health informatics administrative departments or units, usually led by medical doctors with informatics backgrounds.

These informatics departments are responsible for the planning and strategic decisions in relation to informatics, in order to address the needs and demands of the various regional healthcare systems.

HEALTH INFORMATICS CONFIGURATION

The social technical configuration of the Spanish health informatics sector includes a wide range of knowledge producers, technology developers and adapters, and final users. It also is made up of different types of networks that are formulated by the actors who make up the configuration. In this case, the actors identified for this study included firms, hospitals, public administrators, and public/academic researchers related to the field. Following are the main results of our fieldwork aggregated by type of actor.

Firms

In Spain, firms working in areas related to healthcare informatics can actually be grouped into three categories: (1) the more "traditional" in nature—that is, medical informatics firms that provide software and services to the healthcare system; (2) established firms that have always been providers of electromedical equipment and devices to the healthcare sector but recently have integrated information systems; and, finally, (3) the "newcomers," the telecommunication firms, which have no tradition whatsoever in the health sector but have shown interest because of the technological opportunities and future developments in health information and communication technology (ICT).

The firms in Spain that work in the health information technology sector range from multinationals mostly of U.S. origin, such as Hewlett-Packard and SMS, to small specialized firms that provide software systems for niche markets such as Internet services, web pages for medical associations, software providers of pharmaceuticals management within hospitals, and so on. Currently there are several advanced health informatics systems that have been successfully implemented in Spanish hospitals. These include not only EPR but telemedical systems and, in general, the firms believe that there are many examples of technologically advanced hospitals in the Spanish healthcare service that are comparable to other countries in Europe.

Among the firms interviewed, we found that skills and training for human resources were highly valued. There were cases of medical professionals with competencies in informatics as well as telecommunications engineers with experience in the health sector. When firms were too small to have personnel with medical backgrounds, they used expert committees of doctors (direct contacts) for advisory purposes. These firms used expert opinion and advice because they believed that developing ICT systems for hospitals was quite different than developing ICT banking systems, for example. One respondent described a hospital as operating "like a hotel, a catering service, a laboratory, a firm, etc.; it's more than just healing people."

However, interestingly enough, one of the main innovation-management needs expressed by the firms was exactly that, the need for human resources, especially those who were familiar with the healthcare sector (medical or biological backgrounds) and also had training and skills in telecommunication and information technologies. The innovation management resource needs focused mostly on this aspect, the human factor, and less on financial, technical, or knowledge needs.

In addition, firms interviewed indicated that the structural changes mentioned above in centralized decision making for health informatics had not significantly affected the relationship between suppliers of technology (firms) and final consumers (hospital or primary care center). Although decisions were made at the centralized level, firms stated that they still needed to approach hospital directors and medical professionals to present new technologies and use bottom-up sales and marketing strategies before getting approval to enter the public healthcare system.

Future expectations in the firms' perspective for the development of information technologies in the Spanish health sector include the integration of primary and secondary care, which would be achieved by both EPR and telemedical systems. However, the main obstacles for these developments, in their opinion, were medical professionals and their resistance to change in working structures and organizational aspects.

Hospitals

In Spain, hospital information systems have evolved from those implemented for administrative and managerial purposes to also include applications that have more clinical and diagnostic applications linked directly to patient care. This has its roots in the idea that health informatics can no longer be considered a tool that simply permits improved organization for optimizing resources, improving storage and scheduling, and so forth but rather as a strategic element that is essential for increased quality in overall patient care service and provision. Consequently, informatics is evolving from isolated computer applications within a hospital unit to integrated information technology systems within units, between them, and throughout the healthcare service. For example, INSALUD is currently implementing an intranet among close to 100 hospitals for data and information exchange.

All the INSALUD hospitals operate with basic hospital information systems. These systems are the first of several building blocks for technological advances toward EPR. The innovation strategies of firms in Spain have been to develop modular systems—that is, components that can be built on, or added to, once the main infrastructure is set up. This offers many advantages and allows for customization. As for specific initiatives in EPR, two examples are the relatively new hospitals (created in 1997) that have advanced informatics systems. These are the Fundación Hospital Alcorcón in Madrid (a public foundation) and the Hospital de la Ribera de Alzira in Valencia (private management for public service), which claim to be "paperless" hospitals.

Besides these two new hospitals, there are hospitals in other parts of Spain that have adopted EPR systems, partially eliminating physical paper support for patient records [6]. In addition, some hospitals have set up research departments that are exclusively dedicated to research and development projects that in many cases are related to information technology and bioengineering. These research groups often contract telecommunication engineers who also have background in the biological sciences. These groups conduct pilot projects in many fields and develop sophisticated software systems with the aim of solving specific problems in other medical areas.

The main future expectations for those interviewed are the widespread use of the Internet, the integration of primary and secondary care, and the development of an interoperatable electronic patient record (full integration and exchange) among healthcare services, as well as telemedical applications, especially geared toward home monitoring and telediagnostics. The perceived barrier to these developments is the medical professional who needs to be better trained to use these technologies.

Public Management Organizations

Regulation and data protection of patient data are controlled by the Data Protection Agency and administrative departments within the Ministry of Health, such as the Sub-Directorate General for Information Technology Systems. In addition, INSALUD has an Organization and Planning Department, which coordinates and manages issues related to the application of new technologies. These administrative bodies play an important role in the adoption and implementation of EPR systems and, when interviewed, were very optimistic about the development of these systems in Spanish hospitals.

There are also medical technology evaluation agencies that serve as consultative and advisory bodies and produce periodic reports evaluating and assessing new medical technologies. Currently, there are three agencies in Spain: the National Medical Technology Evaluation Agency (a national level agency that is a part of the Carlos III Health Institute and is directly linked to the Ministry of Health) and two regional agencies—the Catalonian Healthcare Service (Barcelona) and the Andalusian Healthcare Service (Seville). However, the relationship between the public healthcare service and these agencies has been characterized as an instrument for the cost-containment concerns that public officials have due to the increasing costs of medical technology.

In this sense we cannot ignore the role played by intermediate organizations such as consulting firms and technology assessment agencies, which influence the decision-making system with studies and reports commissioned by healthcare officials. These intermediate actors make judgments and evaluations on technological innovations that set scenarios for how the hospital of the future will look.

The expectations among public administrators who were interviewed coincided with the other actors—that is, the integration of primary care and hospitals to achieve improved healthcare provision for citizens. In addition, they mentioned the use of information technologies to help contain cost and improve efficiency, and the use of decision support systems. Again, the main problem is the need for continued training of medical professionals in the area of informatics and a reduction in their resistance to change current work practices.

Public Research Organizations and Universities

Several research organizations and university groups develop software systems for medical professionals and new technologies in health informatics. The groups range from those that are very international—that is, highly involved in European Union–funded research projects working with other university groups or hospitals outside of Spain—to those that are locally focused. The locally funded groups work more directly with the Spanish medical profession to solve their problems in relation to information management and knowledge sourcing by developing decision support systems, access to databases, medical protocol guides, and so forth, or by setting up training courses and information dissemination tools. Some groups are linked to telecommunication faculties and have a more telemedicine or bioengineering focus, while those linked to informatics faculties and/or artificial intelligence departments follow other types of research and development lines. The directors of these groups often have combined backgrounds in informatics and medicine. As are other research groups in Spain, these organizations are highly dependent on public funding for their research and development activities.

Of the groups interviewed, scenarios for future development include paperless hospitals as well as robotically and electronically controlled operating rooms. EPR was seen as an essential system not only to integrate the healthcare service but also as a means of obtaining valuable information for research and development (epidemiological studies, public health, etc.). The medical profession was again viewed as a problem, although these groups also mentioned the lack of strategic planning on behalf of the healthcare services in the adoption of telematic systems for hospitals.

CONFIGURATION DYNAMICS AND EPR

The most notable result found in our analysis was the convergence of expectations centered on the development of EPR. The majority of the actors interviewed mentioned the importance of EPR systems in Spanish healthcare service. In addition, and highly related to EPR, most people believed it was quite important to connect primary and secondary care, and they saw the future moving toward a more integrated system, in particular through the use of telemedicine (teleradiology, telediagnostics) and the use of an interoperatable electronic patient record. The future scenario for healthcare service was characterized as an intranet of the various primary healthcare centers and their corresponding hospitals and, eventually, intercommunication existing between and among hospitals. We should note that in no case was there reference to a unified EPR (i.e., for all of Spain) among the regional healthcare services. At most, the importance was on information integration and exchange among the healthcare regions.

With respect to innovation management, our study analyzed the organizational level (within the organizations or groups). At this level, we looked at those techniques, skills, and capacities related to managing innovation. Here, our study shows that most actors use knowledge-sourcing techniques for obtaining new ideas and learning about new technology (through technical journals, Internet, etc.) as well as through contacts with experts at seminars and conferences. In large firms, innovation management included market and prospective studies which, in many cases, would come directly from headquarters outside of Spain. Public actors used strategic plans to define priorities for periods of time (either one- or four-year plans) and to coordinate their activities. Research groups managed innovation by exploiting their capacities and also by exploring new ideas, although these were often restricted to the available public funding where priority setting in R&D depends more on this funding than the priorities defined by the funding agencies.

Hospitals, in many cases, needed to establish formalized practices for innovation management, especially with regard to future development for information systems. In the development and definition process involved in creating the new hospitals, groups of individuals representing public officials, firms, and medical professionals were brought together to define the future hospital and to align their preferences and expectations.

Our study shows that most actors identify the lack of human resources as the main barrier to innovation management. Financial resources were also considered important (although that is closely linked to the first one), especially in the case of academic research groups that are highly dependent on external and competitive sources of funding.

It is very evident that HIS (hospital information systems) changes the manner in which doctors, nurses, and other professionals in the hospital work, and this is exactly the problem. In general, the actors interviewed felt that there is a lack of organization within the hospitals and a lack of coordination among the various service units. Another common barrier to the future development of EPR perceived by most of those addressed in this study was the lack of training of healthcare professionals in informatics (although, of course, there are many exceptions, especially in the younger generation) and their resistance to changing their work practices (this ties directly to pressures that come from labor unions, which are quite strong in this sector).

Other obstacles perceived by the actors were the budgetary constraints and bureaucracy involved in purchasing and introducing new technologies into the healthcare system. Nevertheless, a very dynamic relationship emerged among the different types of actors that centers around the Spanish Society of Health Informatics (SEIS), whose executive committee includes medical doctors in hospitals and public researchers from both public research centers and universities.

The mission of the SEIS association is to encourage the utilization of informatics in the area of medicine and health, and to promote advances and research in this area. SEIS publishes bimonthly *I+S Informática y Salud* (Informatics and Health), a magazine aimed at medical professionals, which serves to disseminate information of relative importance in the area of health informatics. It organizes two important biannual conventions (INFOMED and INFOSALUD) that bring together those involved with health informatics. INFOMED is directed mainly at doctors (and firms) and concentrates on areas related to medical informatics (diagnostics, hospital administration and management, patient care, etc.). INFOSALUD is more general (*salud* means health) and is directed to all healthcare professionals, covering a much wider area of "health" (consumer information, pharmaceuticals, education and training, etc).

In addition, SEIS organizes conventions, which are more focused, such as INFOFARMA for the pharmaceutical industry and INFOENFERMERIA for nursing. SEIS also organizes annual debates on the future of specific issues, including current obstacles that impede change, future major impacts that are expected or desired in specific areas, and which ICTs will be crucial to make them possible.

The interactions among actors depend somewhat on important informal ties (personal contacts and friendships) that have developed over time because the same people are moving within these organizational settings (among firms, public administration, and research groups).

The Spanish case for EPR illustrates how global expectations of future development in the areas of health informatics have been successfully translated into localized initiatives and innovative strategies to promote healthcare delivery in the Spanish healthcare system. This configuration, although constrained by institutional arrangements in the healthcare system through initiatives primarily organized by the Spanish Health Informatics Society, has prioritized the importance of telemedical systems and EPR in Spanish hospitals.

The dynamics of both configurations—telemedicine and EPR in Spain—can be characterized by a clear supplier-client relationship between firms and hospitals as well as by a financial resource dependency of the R&D actors on public funds for innovation and technology development. The firms' ability to produce, develop, and sell depend on public healthcare budgets that designate (often restricted) amounts for purchasing new technologies and, as a result, technological adoption and diffusion are dependent on the national healthcare system. The research groups obtain funds for their R&D projects through public research programs that follow priorities set at the national level. Consequently, it is well recognized that the development of the healthcare informatics sector is highly dependent on the public sector, which thus gives it a privileged position to enhance or inhibit the development and diffusion of new technologies. Both configurations exhibit high resource dependencies as well as strong binding rules that constrain or enhance their activities.

The dynamics of expectations that mobilize actors in different directions depend on their interactions, which either encourage or inhibit adoption and diffusion of technology, where these interactions rely on both formal and informal linkages. As a result, we witnessed pressure from hospitals on regional healthcare services concerning their demands and their needs. Second, firms use their marketing strategies to introduce innovations by creating the demand (convincing hospital directors and healthcare professionals of their needs). Next, we have public researchers and academics who are in contact with other actors outside of Spain, bringing in promises and expectations from the international context. For example, actors consider EPR as something that is necessary (and inevitable), and since they perceive that other countries are already moving in that direction, they believe that Spain should too. The promise is that EPR will help healthcare delivery. International expectations are adopted (and adapted) at the local level—that is, each hospital tries to move closer in that direction (many EPR-type initiatives in hospitals all over Spain).

The general discourse centers on the need to integrate primary and secondary care more effectively, based on scenarios built around telemedicine and EPR. Actors see telemedicine techniques as connecting primary healthcare centers to hospitals (to reduce overload in hospitals, to avoid unnecessary movement of elderly patients, or in low density regions, employing telediagnostics, telemonitoring, specialized teleradiology, cardiology, etc.) and the use of EPR as reducing paperload and increasing/improving accessibility throughout the hospital or even in the primary care center.

Many of the activities organized by SEIS have brought together actors from both primary and secondary care. The need to improve communication and set long-term commitments has brought optimism to the healthcare delivery in many local healthcare areas. SEIS has been a key actor in the general dynamics of the configuration by mobilizing and enrolling the actors to share promises and expectations in the development of the healthcare sector in general, with the overall mission to improve and promote healthcare delivery.

In summary, scenarios are built and expectations are created as a result of the interactions among the actors in the configuration where coordination and priority setting are mediated by SEIS through information exchange and interaction among actors. Future developments in healthcare delivery center around integrating and improving the connection between primary and secondary care through information and communication technologies applied to the health sector. Still, the "passage" point for all these developments depends highly on the healthcare services. Although they have recently increased their budgets in investments for new technology, there still is a long way to go.

FINAL REMARKS

Although our discourse has been on integration of the healthcare system, the underlying dynamics is reasoning or matching needs with opportunities. These configurations are built on resource dependencies controlled by the national healthcare service, whose main concern is to promote healthcare while reducing and controlling increasing costs. The opportunity for health informatics is the promise that these new technologies will provide cost saving through increased efficiency.

The general expectations that center around EPR are a result of international scenarios, promises, and general trends, but the questions we pose are: Why do these expectations become important? And under what conditions do they become influential in the Spanish context? We have found that there is a key role played by the professional association, the Spanish Society for Health Informatics. This institutional actor is an aggregator and coordinator of actors and serves to converge and align expectations. The case of Spain is an example of successful localized initiatives as opposed to the development in other countries toward "the EPR," a single national, centralized, and integrated system.

NOTES

[1] The European Commission has promoted research in this area through Framework Programs such as AIM and Telematics for Healthcare. See CORDIS web page at http://www.cordis.lu/en/home.html.

[2] This chapter is a result of work carried our by the research project entitled FORMAKIN (Foresight as a Tool for Management of Knowledge and Innovation), financed by the European Commission IV Framework Program TSER and the IV National Research Plan. See the web site for Workpackage Reports at http://www.iesam.csic.es/proyecto/formakin.htm.

[3] Spain has a decentralized national healthcare service, the largest healthcare provider is INSALUD which serves 60 percent of the population in 10 regions, while the rest of the seven autonomous regions have competencies in health care and have set up regional services. The future healthcare policy is for all regions to have competencies in healthcare provision.

[4] For more details, see A. Rico, "Regional Decentralization and Health Care Reform in Spain (1976–1996)" in *Comparing Social Welfare Systems in Southern Europe*, Florence Conference, Vol. 3 (1997), pp. 201–228.

[5] See Final Report Part 7 Annexes to the Final Report of FORMAKIN (Country Case Studies) at http://www.york.ac.uk/org/satsu/OnLinePapers/Online Papers.htm.

[6] Two examples are the relatively new hospitals, the Fundación Hospital Alcorcón (Madrid) and Hospital de la Ribera Alzira (Valencia), which claim to be paperless and also have other advanced multimedic clinical and diagnostic systems.

Chapter 4

National Culture and the Design of Medical Technology

Christopher M. Barlow

It has long been understood that people of different national cultures can think about the same thing in quite different ways. Science and engineering have worked hard to develop methods for assessing the universal truths of various phenomena or designs, often determining that various "truths" passed on socially or through national folklore are incorrect. When the truth of some phenomena is defined down to the readings on some meters in a clear protocol, researchers and designers around the world tend to get the same answer. As long as engineering and science discussions focus on elements for which there are clear protocols and metrics, consensus on decision making is fairly easy. However, technology is not a success until it fits the people that will select it, operate it, and use it. As science and engineering attempt to convert technical discoveries into technologies, devices, and systems that provide benefits worth their cost, culture-based differences in belief, behavior, relationships, and thinking style can have profound impacts on the benefits and costs of any particular design. It is likely that the world will reap the greatest benefits of health-related technology from those designers who understand how culture impacts their design efforts, the selection of technology, the use of technology, and how it determines even the very definition of health.

BELIEF AND SCIENCE

Science has always seen itself as rising above superstition and socially constructed beliefs, with few admitting the obvious fact that opinion puts filters on what scientists can begin to research or be funded to research.

Koestler [1] points out that at one time any scientist who sought to study meteors was considered insane. Everybody knew that rocks could not fall from the sky. Those who reported seeing such things were labeled as mental defectives or liars (identical to our reactions to those who claim to experience or research contacts with extraterrestrials). Then, in 1776, a large meteor shower in France was seen by everyone in a respectable town, including the doctors and the police and the priests and the mayor. Suddenly society changed its belief and meteors could be researched.

One of the sad times of medicine was when women were frequently dying soon after childbirth from "puerperal fever." Doctors refused to consider that they were killing the women with their lack of handwashing. More recently, pharmaceutical firms invested millions in acid-conquering drugs for ulcers, seeing a great market in overstressed managers with ulcers and medical plans. Apparently they ignored what veterinarians had known for years—when something gets ulcers, an antibiotic clears it up. The phenomenon was finally confirmed in humans, so now the pharmaceutical companies resort to consumer advertising to sell their "wonder drugs" as a way for people to eat foods like chili and pizza that might otherwise upset their stomachs.

Many doctors, firm in their education, loudly denounce people exploring alternatives to pharmacy and surgery as being unscientific and untested by double-blind studies, when many of their most effective medicines are high-volume copies of herbal medicines, and when many of their methods, such as chemotherapy, have never been subject to double-blind studies. Some of these same doctors use powerful medicines with proven dangerous side effects because they have been assured that the side effects never really happen and don't really cause all that much trouble when they do.

According to Weinberg [2], most fish that have the ability to generate light were discovered about the same time period, except one which was discovered decades later because it uses its light-emitting ability in the daytime not at night, when the scientists were looking for light-emitting fish.

It is critical to utilize the methods of science and technology to clarify as many truths as possible, but it is also critical to recognize that before the science is applied, politics and social beliefs have restricted the truths that can be looked at. Further, in the study of health, disease, and medicine, different cultures can set very different playing fields.

MEDICINE AND CULTURE

Payer and White [3] make a strong case that beliefs about diseases and cures are strongly affected by cultural backgrounds—and not just between the modern doctor and the Third World witch-doctor but also among First World countries such as the United States, England, and Germany. There are quite different attitudes toward what health is, different beliefs of where diseases reside, different beliefs about what to do about disease, and different beliefs about what is an acceptable side effect.

Lorig [4] discusses a growing tendency to shift from a model of an ignorant patient helped by expert doctor to a concept of an intelligent patient who works collaboratively with the doctor to address medical issues. One large and growing market for medical technology consists of these "intelligent" patients who are willing and able to pay for medical devices they can use at home, at work, and throughout their day to monitor important metrics. Diabetics can already routinely monitor their blood sugar levels, and similar devices are being purchased to allow home monitoring of levels of blood thinners and other health-related measures.

The growing "alternative" or "complementary" health cultures seem eager to acquire technology that guides them as they use nonpharmaceutical approaches to reduce blood pressure, cholesterol, and other threats to heart and blood vessel function. As other tests of blood chemistry and body processes become available, patients can constantly adjust to maximize effectiveness of their health-building activities while minimizing negative side effects.

The cultural assumptions of medical technology firms and design teams can prevent them from recognizing large areas of opportunity that can not only build organizational health but fund continuing development. Deliberate efforts to expose key decision makers and key creators to the multiple mindsets of the patients and healthcare deliverers of the areas they would like to impact can greatly increase organizational success. It can also result in designs whose better fit to the culture means greater health impact.

It is important to note that there is an essential difference between the economic realities of medical practitioners and medical technology producers. A practitioner well enmeshed in the local cultural assumptions about medicine can have a long and prosperous practice, regardless of the beliefs and practices of other cultures. However, medical technology can generally reap the benefits of economies of scale. Products or services that attract well-funded users beyond the limits of a particular culture result in production volumes that quickly bring the costs down, thus extending the health benefits to far more people while generating larger cash flows to fund more interesting research. If your competitor outreaches you, it is hard to stay in existence.

Cognitive Complexity and Cultural Knowledge/Beliefs

It is easy to say that people should understand and accept the cultural values and beliefs of others, but people vary in their ability to simultaneously process conflicting beliefs. This is a dimension that psychologists label "cognitive complexity." Those lower in this dimension have difficulty with conflicting beliefs and are more responsive to a process called "cognitive dissonance" in which people shift their beliefs to get them to be more congruent. If a person we like has an opinion we do not like, those lower in cognitive complexity either reduce their liking of the person or increase their acceptance of the opinion.

Cultures make distinctions that are absolute, often tacitly held truths, and therefore difficult to question. Food is a great example. There is little in biology to eliminate most possible foods from the human diet, but cultures make a great distinction between what is and is not food. As an American, I was astonished when a colleague from Czechoslovakia refused my offer of a slice of that great American favorite, pumpkin pie, because in her country pumpkin was fed to pigs, not people. My American students have a hard time understanding how Hindu students could turn down a cheeseburger, but the American would be shocked if offered a horsemeat sandwich. In our minds, whether a cow or a dog or a pumpkin is people food is an absolute truth. Culturally learned truths about medicine, science, and technology are just as absolute, and often have as little validity.

This does not mean that I must accept and adopt the beliefs of other cultures or be tolerant of their intolerance. If I want to host people from many cultures, it is not necessary that I join them in their beliefs, but it is helpful if I am aware of their beliefs and maintain respect for their desires. This does not mean that I am going to serve horse or dog at my picnic but that I am not going to have a pig on a spit when I invite over those who would be offended. If a guest is from a culture that expects women or people of a certain background to be subservient or invisible, I am going to explain that other cultures get respect, not obedience.

In the same way, as medical technology develops, it is important that designers and decision makers are aware of and comprehend the culture-based "truths" of customers and healthcare deliverers. This often requires increased cognitive complexity on their part. While some may simply be incapable of this diverse perspective, many have had their perspective limited by their cultural setting and life history but have the mental capacity for cognitive complexity once they have some enlightening experiences.

The Challenge of Teams

Science and/or design efforts reflecting the breadth of relevant technical knowledge as well as the breadth of issues impacting those involved in health are beyond the scope of knowledge and capacity of any one individual. This leads to the requirement for collaborative efforts by people of diverse backgrounds and knowledge, whether in structured organizations, cross-functional teams, or simply passing subsolutions to others in the marketplace. Of course, collaboration and teamwork actually conflict with the cultural assumptions of some, but most successful science and design supporting organizations recognize the value of well-managed teamwork and collaboration.

To deal with reality effectively, these collaborations consist of people from a great variety of disciplines and knowledge bases. Researchers in teamwork have long understood the importance of trust in team effectiveness, but these "cross-functional" teams have a special aspect that interferes with trust building. A great deal of research has been based on sports teams or work teams. In these teams, the competence of the various team members is obvious very quickly. However, in cross-functional teams, because the various team members come from different disciplines and knowledge domains, they cannot assess the quality of work of their colleagues. An accountant is unlikely to be able to check the calculations and logic of the engineer and thereby know to what degree the person's engineering competence should be trusted.

Therefore, in these teams, trust can only be built personally, in social ways that allow each team member to assess the character and integrity of other team members, to decide whether to allow each of the other team members to influence the team member's thinking. This is a difficult task in any team, but most teams attacking complex issues such as medical technology draw their members from many different cultures. These cultures may provide quite different "truths" about who to trust, how to work with others, and how to organize creative work, as well as different views on health and health care.

Culture Styles of Hofstede

One of the more interesting writers about cultural differences in thinking and values is Geert Hofstede [5], who gathered data from managers in a large technically oriented multinational company. The managers were very similar in jobs and training but represented most of the cultures of the world. He found that along four dimensions, people of the same culture were more like each other and different from other cultures. More recent work to include Chinese managers has led to a fifth factor.

Note that these are not types, but rather ranges across which people are positioned, with different averages for each culture. Note that since we are discussing the average, the central tendency for each culture, there are many individuals in any one culture who are closer to the average of another culture than to their own.

Power Distance

Some people are more comfortable with hierarchy and authority relationships. In countries such as Malaysia and Guatemala, people find it normal for someone to have a great deal more or less power than they do. In countries at the other end of the spectrum, such as Israel and Austria, it is very uncomfortable to have anyone in authority over you. The United States scores 40 on his standardized 100-point scale, leaning toward less acceptance of authoritarian relationships. Note that this factor is not one's need to be high in a hierarchy. Both those who accept being on the lower rungs of society and those who feel they have been born to rule are high on this dimension.

Individualism/Collectivism

Ties are weaker between members of more individualist societies such as the United States and Australia. People are expected to take care of themselves and not rely upon others. In more collectivist societies like Ecuador and Guatemala, people have strong ties with family, village, society, and so forth, and success of the whole is far more important than the success of any one member. People from a collectivist culture see teams as a great chance to work with and help each other. Americans tend to value teams where they can best show off their abilities.

Uncertainty Avoidance

People differ in the degree to which they feel threatened by uncertainty. Those from cultures high in uncertainty avoidance, like Portugal and Greece, take strong steps to increase predictability, often with written and unwritten rules everyone must follow. Those low in uncertainty avoidance, such as Jamaica, are far more comfortable with change, even when they cannot reliably predict the results of the change. The United States leans toward less uncertainty avoidance, scoring an index of 46 out of 100.

Masculine/Feminine

This factor has nothing to do with sexual preference. Hofstede has labeled as masculine those cultures in which there is a strong distinction between the task-oriented male role and the nurturing female role, such as Japan and Austria. He has labeled as feminine those societies in which men and women are equally willing to be strong and nurturing, such as Norway and Sweden. The United States leans more toward the masculine with an index of 62 out of 100.

Time Horizon

In his more recent writings, Hofstede has been exploring the fit of these factors to the Chinese and other Asian cultures not included in his original sample. In addition to the four factors mentioned above, he is looking at a dimension he discusses in terms of Confucian values, but which seems strongly similar to the time horizon factor of Elliott Jaques [6]. Some people tend to consider only the immediate impact of ideas and decisions, while others look far into the future. Jaques has found that generally the higher a person is in an organization, the further they are looking into the future. It is obvious that cultures also differ in their focus on the future. Some only consider today, while others consider generations far into the future.

REAL WORLD IMPLICATIONS: THE "GLOBAL"

Some people learn of these differences and attempt to apply these population averages to individuals, often with strange results. I am aware of a recent joint engineering project between a Japanese and an American manufacturer. After intensive "multicultural training," the engineers met for the first time. The Americans entered bowing and holding out their business cards, while the Japanese greeted them with a big hello and a hearty handshake. They had been trained to be each other.

People diverge from the average, so the individual you are thinking about might actually be far from the average. This is especially likely for people who have moved out of their country for school or work. Basically, if they were close to their home values, they would still be there. International travel seems more likely among those who feel at odds with their home culture, so an individual is less likely to match those still at home.

Another process takes place with travel and experience. Many people become what might best be described as a "global." They are aware of the breadth of cultural differences and prepared to cope with them. Their style is likely to deviate from the home culture, and they are more able to work with people of different styles.

Of course, even when team members do not match their home culture or when all the team members come from the same background, there is generally going to be variation along the five dimensions within the team.

Design Team Dynamics

It should be readily apparent that people differing on these dimensions will be challenged when attempting effective collaboration. High power-distance people try to get the hierarchy established, while low power-distance people try to avoid any such structure. High uncertainty-avoidance people try to move fast to get decisions made and to clarify specifications, while low uncertainty-avoidance team members are trying to keep the limitations on their thinking open as long as possible. What is very interesting about these dimensions and differences is that these are identical to the factors that process facilitators try to manage when trying to maximize the effectiveness of teams and design projects.

Brainstorming as a Culture Shift

Alex Osborn was an advertising executive who noticed that junior people with interesting ideas were not saying them in the meetings. He realized that the usual meeting environment discouraged people from both flexibility and fluency, so he designed a meeting environment called brainstorming to get the creative ideas out for discussion.

He realized that people kept silent because of their fear of the opinions and criticisms of others. With Osborn's four basic rules, groups were able to work together and generate 50 to 500 ideas in five minutes. His groups were so productive that no secretary could keep up, so sessions were tape-recorded, and typed transcripts were given to those attending for later evaluation.

Osborn's brainstorming technique can be seen first as a call to reduce people's avoidance of uncertainty. They were encouraged to contribute ideas of which they were not certain. It was also as a request for people to reduce their power distance. People were encouraged to contribute ideas that conflicted with those of their boss and those of people with more credentials in a discipline.

It is important to note that brainstorming only works on people who need it. Its success depends on the team members' acceptance of the power distance of the facilitator, on the certainty given by the guarantee to judge the ideas very carefully later, and by the individual goal of generating ideas high in quantity and diversity. The people we label as "creative" rarely follow the rules of brainstorming. They judge constantly, refuse to listen to the facilitator, and so on. Like judo, the best facilitation techniques use the energy of the tendency they are trying to overcome to beat it.

Many other facilitative approaches can be seen as movements along Hofstede's cultural dimensions. When people are taught to solve problems in teams, they are often encouraged to define the problem in broader terms, considering who else might be affected (being more collective) and how it might affect the future (extending the time horizon). In addition, a great many techniques of "facilitation" of team creativity are more of a nurturing type, affecting the social and emotional interactions of the team members. To deal with these issues simultaneously with task issues requires a move more toward what Hofstede calls the feminine. Again, facilitative techniques work by plugging into cultural values to shift behavior to a type that is normally blocked by cultural values. This goal is based on the assumption that different ideas are available to people of different styles, so creativity consists of looking where you have not already looked, in the place that is not "normal" or "habitual."

Of course, if different cultures are positioned at different points on the dimensions, the direction they need to go to these "hidden" possibilities might be quite different, and the techniques would have to be anchored in their own cultural styles. It leads one to question whether techniques invented for American managers and engineers are the optimum choice for teams from other backgrounds.

American Style Problem Solving?

It may be fair to say that most of the techniques used for team leadership and deliberate creativity are attempts to shift, at least temporarily, away from the more usual American style. They seek to reduce the power distance, decrease the avoidance of uncertainty, extend the time horizon, take a more collective view of success, and utilize the nurturing skills of a "feminine" society.

How effective are the techniques with people from cultures that are already different from the American style? It may be that they are already "creative," or it may be that creativity actually lies in exploring the areas outside one's habitual thinking. So maybe creativity for a Jamaican is to be a little less tolerant of uncertainty, and so on.

Leading Multicultural Teams

If the different types of thinking and discussion that make up effective problem solving are similar to cultural differences, it would seem that the solution is to select people of the right mix of cultures for each team. However, of course, the real issue is what styles they can deliberately adapt together. Let's all be Jamaican for some brainstorming, now be Austrian for idea evaluation, and so forth.

It seems likely that people of different cultures will react differently to the various components of facilitation and leadership attempts. Some will love one part of the process, others will love another. However, if the techniques rely upon American cultural habits for their power, these methods are unlikely to be effective with those of different habits.

Therefore, it seems critical for anyone attempting to lead deliberate creativity by teams to have an understanding of the ways that team members differ. It is also important to understand both the effects and the anchors of various methods and be prepared to design and use methods with different effects and anchors with people whose styles are different.

It is probably even more useful if the team members understand the issues and differences so that they can make adjustments to one another's perspectives and values. When team members understand and are able to discuss their differences in style, culture, and personality, it becomes possible for each team member to participate more effectively in each different aspect of the creative and problem-solving processes.

Designing and Managing a Collaborative Team for Medical Technology

A team assembled to develop a product or service of medical benefit should not only include competence in the various technical fields of knowledge relevant to the problem and solution but also awareness of the values and paradigms of those people involved in utilizing the technology.

Almost inevitably, that team is going to be multicultural, so it is critical that members are flexible and have adequate cognitive complexity to manage conflicting values and thoughts during the design process. It seems very likely that the same flexibility that allows one to work effectively with people of different cultural assumptions is the flexibility that allows a team to discover the most creative and advantageous design possibilities.

Team cohesiveness is not designed and managed like assembling a fine watch; it is a process in which the team members create their own compromises, their own team culture. The friendships, trust, and respectful relationships that arise among the team members are unique to that team and must be developed by the team as it watches itself proceed.

As for process for the team, one model might be to do both ends of each of Hofstede's dimensions, a sort of yin/yang as appropriate to the situation. Therefore, the team gives high power distance to the expertise of people talking in their own knowledge domain, but totally equal on synergy issues and team management. The team might be high in uncertainty avoidance on key issues like schedules and quality and remain as open as long as possible on design features. The team might check to make sure that the product makes strong contributions to health of the patient in the short term and the long term. Certain team members might focus on task, while others focus on social process of the team (masculine style) and while everyone is aware that both task and process need to be supported by everyone (feminine style). And each team member would strive for individual excellence in the part they contribute, while working to make sure the issues brought forward by the many different team members are handled well and the team is a success as a whole.

CONCLUSION

Dynamics of culture, including those of national origin, have a great deal to do with the relative success of different design efforts in medical technology. It would seem that organizers and leaders of these efforts would benefit greatly from understanding cultural differences and dynamics and from helping the design collaborations understand and manage the cultural dynamics of the teams and their interactions.

NOTES

[1] Koestler, A., *Janus* (New York: Random House, 1978).

[2] Weinberg, G. M., *On the Design of Stable Systems* (New York: Wiley Interscience, 1979).

[3] Payer, L., and K. L. White, *Medicine and Culture: Varieties of Treatment in the United States, England, West Germany, and France* (New York: Owlet, 1996).

[4] Lorig, K., "Partnership between Expert Patients and Physicians," *The Lancet*, 359, March 9, 2002, pp. 361–385.

[5] Hofstede, G., *Cultures and Organizations: Software of the Mind* (New York: McGraw-Hill Professional Publishing, 1996).

[6] Jaques, E., *A General Theory of Bureaucracy* (Portsmouth, NH: Heinemann Educational Books, 1976).

Part II

Future Processes of Healthcare Delivery

Chapter 5

Following and Accelerating the Design Evolution Curve in Health Care

Christopher M. Barlow

Health may be the most complex and complicated problem the species has ever worked on, and one certainly high in importance. The human body is certainly very complicated in its composition, dynamics, conflicts, and interactions. The natural environment, which supports and affects human health, is complicated in its composition, dynamics, conflicts, and interactions. The variety of resources developed for increasing human health are certainly complicated in their composition, dynamics, conflicts, and interactions.

The nature of the situation is far out on the dimension of simple to contingent to systematic to heuristic to ecological to chaotic.

Just to make it more interesting, the stakeholders and actors in the situation vary widely in values, goals, and motivations (even within themselves), producing the kind of problem that is labeled "wicked" and requiring the kind of thinking that psychologists label "cognitive complexity," the ability to deal with conflicting values without choosing between them.

Thinking about this complexity could cause one to give up, or to focus just on a perspective of limited complicatedness and complexity, and hope that it works in the world of markets and systemic chaotic interactions. (This limited perspective is the fundamental reality of academic disciplines and functional departments, and the source of their effectiveness.)

It is possible for knowledgeable people from differing perspectives to come together and develop a shared understanding (while their own perspectives, goals, and values remain conflicted) and invent and explore new alternatives that increase the effectiveness of the healthcare system

while maintaining the effectiveness and prosperity of its constituent organizations. The best efforts can leapfrog years of "evolutionary" development and adoption.

Of course, it is difficult for these groups to work together at the highest
level of synergy, especially when there are great differences in technical
field, national origins, and/or cognitive style. Research into complex
problem solving has demonstrated that different approaches to working
together can have quite different levels of effectiveness.

Effective leaders of such efforts have learned to build a different climate of interaction that accepts and values disagreements without re-
solving them early and to build relationships among the participants that
can keep them thinking together while thinking differently. They have
learned to disconnect intention from tradition, asking questions like,
"What does a hospital really do?" and "What else (especially in new
technology) can do that?"

Once the group has begun to accept disagreements and to disconnect
desired benefits from the traditional methods, they are ready to use
methods such as criteria decision matrices and systems models to integrate and synergize their thinking and to use techniques such as analo-
gies and visual brainstorming to generate ideas of sufficient complexity
to meet the realities of the healthcare system.

Such groups can more rapidly see the potentials and problems of such
innovations as a home blood test kit, Internet connections to medical
knowledge and advice, a better educated population, or discovering an
unpatentable cure for a condition that currently generates huge profits
for various players. The quality of their interaction directly affects the
rate of increase in the quality of health in the population and the quality
of health care, so deliberate intervention in the quality of their work has
a direct effect on the performance of the hospital and healthcare system
of the future.

THE NEED FOR DELIBERATE MANAGEMENT OF
COMPLEX CREATIVITY

Although focusing one's creativity and thinking within a perspective
of limited complicatedness and complexity allows some amazing inventions, members of particular disciplines often laugh bitterly at what they
see as the stupidity of humanity, telling stories of "inferior" technologies
dominating the market and of "great" ideas getting rejected. Even ideas
can be widely accepted for their benefit to the players' economics, but
with negative impacts upon actual health of people.

It is easy to blame such failures on the stupidity of others, but is a
technology truly superior if it has characteristics that make it a market
failure, social failure, or ethical failure? Are designers right to believe

that it is impossible to develop inventions that are superior both in technology and in acceptance? What do designers have to do differently if they decide to take responsibility for making new technology a total success?

This chapter explores some famous "mis-designs," considers their causes and how to avoid them, and suggests ways to better address the opportunities available in the health field. Ironically, it can be the very creativity and genius of people who understand a limited part of the problem that leads to some of the biggest problems, a process referred to often in the systems literature as suboptimization. And the real trick to better design is to truly listen to those who resist your ideas. This is a difficult lesson to learn.

Over time, designs improve in a process often called evolution. Like biological evolution, variations on the original emerge. Where biological evolutionary success basically is determined by whether you have more grandchildren than others, in products the issue is the marketplace: Do people make and buy products and services that include your design features? Some features gain support and become part of the product or service; other features find little support and disappear from the most commonly available products.

The evolutionary perspective gives important insights. Neither evolution nor the market always picks the survivors you would like. Mosquitoes continue to survive and evolve no matter how irritating they are to other species. And some products that succeed in the marketplace simply baffle most people (for example, take a look at the other magazines available where you buy yours). Also, many species of animals and plants have evolved as interactive systems in which the new features of one enable the new features of another. In the same way, one technology change can unleash incredible growth in another by removing a critical constraint.

Basically, products and services are bundles of knowledge accumulated and integrated over time. From the Wright brothers' motorized kites with bicycle controls flown at Kitty Hawk to modern jumbo jets, stealth fighters, and even ultra-light planes, there is a great deal of learning, knowledge, and experience embedded in the designs. The speed at which our technologies can learn determines how fast we get new and better benefits. The question is whether technologists in health care can affect the speed at which product effectiveness and efficiency are achieved in the marketplace.

EXAMPLES OF ERRORS

It may be wrong to label these examples as errors because, in many cases, the design was pure genius given the problem they were focusing on. It is just that other parts of the situation they did not understand prevented complete success, or parts of the situation they did understand changed, and the design became a problem.

Changing Realities and Constraints

Most technology lovers are familiar with the "QWERTY" keyboard, standard on English language computers because it was standard on electric typewriters, because it was standard on manual typewriters as a way to slow down the better typists so they wouldn't jam the keys. This was a great creative solution to the biggest problem of that time. It is hard to sell typewriters if your customers spend a lot of time unjamming the keys. As an additional feature for the salesmen, the designers even shifted a few keys so that the word "typewriter" could be typed very fast alternating between two fingers just on the top line so salesmen could make typing look easy and fast. That idea, so useful then, is wasting an incredible amount of time around the planet as we try to type words on a keyboard designed to slow us down.

And of course it was a stroke of genius to use the YYMMDD format for dates, even better the Julian date of two digits for the years and three digits for which day of the 365 in the year. When the author was programming for the J. C. Penney catalog in 1978, giving every transaction the full four digit year would have required the spending of millions of dollars for additional disk drives. Of course, that great efficiency became the Y2K Bug, with inconceivable amounts of money spent to fix that one field.

But as you look back at these two cases, could those designers have understood the potential problems from their creative ideas and developed new ideas that worked in their situation and in the future? And more importantly, can you avoid being the genius who contributes the next QWERTY or Y2K bug to the future of technology?

And, even more disconcerting, how many absolutely required design elements in our systems are related to the old realities and invalid in the new?

Missing Part of the Problem

Petroski [1] tells of the marvelous Britannia Tubular Bridge built in 1850 over the Menai Strait on the northwest coast of Wales to carry passengers to the port for a Dublin-bound ferry. A wrought-iron tube with the train running on the inside, it was a technological marvel of design and construction, a work of true engineering genius. Only after construction was it discovered that the bridge was unusable. Imagine a black, wrought-iron tube sitting in the hot sun of a summer day, with more sunlight reflected off of the water. Imagine the temperature inside as this wonderful solar collector stores heat. Now, take a wood-fired engine pulling a trainload of passengers through this tube with no ventilation. Imagine the heat, the smoke, the sparks flying from the engine. It could easily be described as hell on earth. Examination of the design notes and specifications shows not a single bit of attention paid to the realities of passenger trains, only wind loads and ocean storms and spans. It was a remarkable solution to the problem as understood, but missed one of the most important parts of the problem.

AVOIDING AND OVERCOMING "ERRORS"

Very few individuals have the breadth of background, knowledge, and relationships to pull off a well-designed technological development. So the trick is in assembling a collaboration that is capable of seeing all the issues and all the possibilities. Let's introduce some key ideas from the field of deliberate creativity.

AHA as Insight Shift

So many different people and events are involved in the development and implementation of any innovation, our old concept of inventors getting great ideas and implementing them seems to miss much of what is happening. Barlow [2] proposes that understanding collaborative creativity is facilitated by defining creativity as the changed perspective of the creator rather than ideas. This "shifted insight" model has its roots in that most subjective and individualistic phenomenon of all, the "AHA" or "Eureka!" experience. Throughout history, various individuals such as Koestler [3] have described this reaction a person has to getting an idea. This intensely physical, emotional, and intellectual experience seems to mark our fundamental recognition that a profoundly advantageous change has taken place in our thinking. Figure 5.1 attempts to explain this model.

1. A flashlight has been chosen for the model as an analogy for our perception of a problem. The surface below represents all the things anyone could ever do. The area of the surface illuminated by a flashlight signifies the set of ideas that fit the problem statement. If the flashlight represents a problem statement or intention like "raise the bridge," the illuminated circle represents all the various actions that might raise the bridge.

2. A second flashlight represents a new formulation of the problem, such as "increase the gap between the bridge and the water" or "get tall boats past the bridge." The surface area that its pool of light illuminates includes all the ways to accomplish that goal. In successful creativity,

Figure 5.1
The Eureka Experience

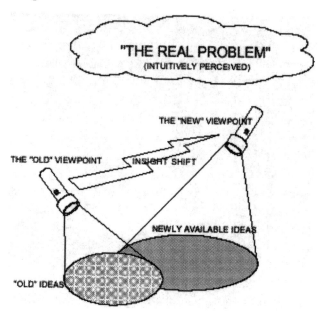

some of the alternatives illuminated or made obvious by this new view-point are better than the best of the ideas made obvious by the old perspective. The advantage of the new perspective can be as profound as shifting your calculations from Roman numerals to Arabic notation. Problems like multiplication and division that are basically impossible in Roman numerals are simple (though sometimes tedious) in the new representation. This shifted perspective can be a simple assumption about the situation or as profound as a basic paradigm of a discipline or culture.

3. The lightning bolt labeled "insight shift" represents the shift to the new definition. Although getting such an insight might take years, when it happens, it seems as fast as that lightning bolt.

4. The cloud above represents the "real" problem, the complex interaction of wants, wishes, and reality that is only approximated by our viewpoints and problem statements. Locating the second flashlight of the new viewpoint closer to that cloud represents our perception of the closer fit of the new perception to the total problem.

Let's discuss some of the implications of this model:

1. The strength of the AHA or Eureka! experience is directly related to the perceiver's image of the problem, not the broad quality of the idea. The better the fit of the perceiver's knowledge to the breadth of

issues involved, the more relevant the AHA response. For example, if we are having a casual conversation with a new acquaintance, and we mention a problem we are facing, that person may get a great AHA reaction to an idea about what we should do, an idea that fits their misunderstanding of the problem. On the other hand, if their comment or idea triggers a shift in our perception to a point that better fits our perception of the problem and makes obvious some new and useful alternatives, our AHA reaction is relevant, especially since we are the ones to act on the new perception.

2. Our AHA response to someone else's idea or suggestion, an "Appreciative AHA," is a measure of the value of that idea or perspective to the problem as we see it. It is entirely possible for a nonexpert to trigger such a response in an expert, a relevant AHA that indicates the potential of an idea, but the relevance of the response depends on the breadth of understanding of the perceiver.

3. It is important to note that the problem as perceived, the context of our AHA reaction, includes our values and wishes as well as our knowledge and experiences. So, for example, if there is a person at work who has really irritated you, and a new perspective or idea occurs to you that not only seems to fit the problem but also really punishes your opponent, your AHA will have more energy. The same is true of your good wishes for others. So if you hate or disrespect your customers, the ideas that really light your fire will be those that punish your customers. For this reason, cross-functional teams that appreciate one another's perspectives, even when they disagree, would seem more likely to get AHAs that meet the needs of more perspectives and stakeholders.

4. Satisficing is another important aspect of this creative process. Simon [4] used the term to describe our tendency to decide to accept less than optimum solutions because the improvement to optimum was not worth the effort to gather and analyze additional data. One of the things that happens to people who participate in an AHA experience is that their expectations and perceptions of the situation change. We often talk of the "Not Invented Here" syndrome because it seems that organizations and departments refuse to accept ideas developed by outsiders, but would accept them if they developed them themselves. Note that after you shift to the new perception, the new ideas seem obvious, but if you are still back at the old perspective, the new ideas are ridiculous. A good example of this phenomenon would be planning a family vacation. If you sat down, gathered all relevant data and effectively planned the absolutely best possible vacation for your family given the conditions, family members would all complain and be dissatisfied because your plan would be pretty poor from their individual perspectives. On the other hand, if they had been in on the planning, the process would have

had an effect on their understanding and expectations, and they would have shifted to a perspective in which your plan is quite good.

So we can see that the knowledge background, beliefs, intentions, and other mental processes all impact individuals' creativity and their reactions to the creativity of others. Deliberate efforts to improve the creative complexity must find ways to impact these factors.

The Curse of Mental Success

One problem faced by many people who have been successful in technical fields is that they always got high grades in school. When they took a test, they rarely made an error. As a result, they have had the consistent experience that every time they felt really good about an idea, the idea was right. Of course, the point they missed was that the tests they took were deliberately designed to be single-domain problems with correct answers. Unfortunately, the real world is full of messy, multiple-domain problems with no single clear answer. With such real-world problems, the poor students have a definite advantage. Throughout their academic career, whenever they felt good about an answer, they were wrong about 35 percent of the time. So they never trust their own judgment and instincts; they check with other people to make sure they understand the full problem and its possible solutions.

Full Spectrum Design

One of the best descriptions for the problem of complete design is the old story of the blind men and the elephant, in which each of the blind men encountered a different part of the elephant, then argued about the true nature of the elephant. What is interesting to note is that each blind man is right about his part, yet wrong in his total perception. Each has had a powerful AHA experience that explains what he knows about the elephant. But until they can let go of their conclusions, share their information, and experiment with different perspectives and models, they cannot understand the elephant.

A great example of dealing with this issue was the design project for the Ford Taurus. Lew Veraldi, leading the project, mapped out every organization and type of individual who had an interest in the final design of the car, whether repair shop mechanics, legislative bodies, or production workers. Each stakeholder group was approached, and a list of their "demands" was created. Each demand was dealt with, although often in a way different from the suggestion. For example, assembly workers demanded that they get rid of plastic bumpers. Instead of accepting the idea, which would have caused real problems in fuel efficiency, the project team asked why. It turned out that the original implementation of plastic bumpers had endcaps to go around the corners of the car that were almost impossible to align. To solve the real problem more completely, they found that they could mold plastic bumpers that would go around the corners, thus keeping the weight down, eliminating the alignment problems, and improving the appearance. They went through all the requests of all the stakeholders and dealt with them in a similar fashion. The resulting design won many awards and captured a very large market share.

Several other cases of team design are given by Nonaka and Takeuchi [5]—for example, the Canon personal copier, bread-making machines, and automobiles. Interestingly, in a time when middle managers are being eliminated from companies and replaced with macros in distributed databases, Nonaka argues that only middle managers are equipped to lead and manage the collaboration among functional departments, which is the knowledge-creating engine of organizations. In the medical and healthcare system, these players probably do not even work for the same organization. Unfortunately, most of these managers have only been trained to act as individual data processing links and, like most engineers, have little preparation for the kinds of leadership and management necessary to make team collaboration effective.

MAKING THE PROCESS WORK BETTER

A manager needs different skills and abilities to deal with this more complex task. For example, one of the key questions in establishing a collaborative design process is how to increase the probability of "Relevant AHAs." How do we make sure that every part of the "elephant" is included in the discussion? One aspect is selection of participants; the other is the guidance of a process in which participants can both affect the discussion with their knowledge and be affected by the discussion, reformulating their own perspective on the problem. It is important to note that for most problems, the players do not all belong to the same department, and often not even to the same corporate organization. It may be useful to partner with customers, suppliers, even competitors and regulators to build a more effective collaboration. Of course, getting them into the room, as hard as it is, is the easy part. Helping the interaction flourish is quite difficult. Because each participant has different perspectives and goals as well as a history of conflict and interaction, creative conversation is often difficult, beyond the skills of most managers. For example, since most have been trained in rational decision making with well-structured problems, they think that all problems are like that. Classic decision making starts with clear agreement upon and consensus about the problem, the facts, and the criteria. But real design problems are ill structured, with constraints and criteria in so many conflicting domains that a clear decision is impossible. And most are actually of the type called "wicked": even when we clearly understand the problem, the players disagree about the ultimate goals and values. Even when the most successful, complex, diverse team has designed and accepted a course of action, there are still strong disagreements about the goals, facts, and criteria. The trick is to work together in relative disagreement, seeking out all the clarifications and simplifications possible, but accepting that consensual clarity is impossible.

Barlow [2] discovered that some techniques seemed to have very strong contributions to these multiperspective design efforts. In this analysis, ideas are seen as more creative when they involve more disciplines or require so much of a shift in the problem definition that the problem must be re-explained to management. One surprise of the research was that ideas that are more creative in this sense are more likely to be accepted by the organization, leading to the possible conclusion that many ideas are rejected simply because they are not creative or complex enough. The strategy of separating the benefits from the attributes and realizing that attributes cost money but customers pay for benefits is extremely powerful. This strategy is often referred to in systems design as "black box" thinking and is called "function analysis" in the field of Value Engineering [6–8]. Even more powerful is a technique where a team analyzes the cost for each increment of benefit the customer is buying as well as the price the customer is willing and able to pay for that increment. [9]

A second technique that is strongly related to creative team success is the use of the criteria decision matrix in which each alternative is evaluated against each criteria. Although these techniques might be seen by many as too confining and analytical to allow creativity, they seemed to lead to a deeper, more complex understanding of the situation, allowing more complexly creative ideas to emerge.

As logical as these approaches seem, it is difficult for most people to shift their perceptions from the tried and true, especially when interacting with others. Building a climate and culture of interaction in a team that allows and encourages people to move away from these more acceptable perceptions can be a very difficult process, but it is possible. There are many resources on teamwork and facilitation that can be helpful here, but it is often possible to find someone trained and experienced in this area to help a team or interaction. Basically, it involves building a culture of trust in which exercising flexibility of thinking is seen as success, not deviance. And the best indicator of the success of such a culture is laughter and good humor as the team plays with various outrageous concepts.

The critical point is that while most engineers and managers are poorly prepared to lead or work in such multiperspective creative teams, it is possible to get more people involved more effectively in design discussions, developing designs that normally might have taken several market cycles to correct.

OTHER PERSPECTIVES TO SATISFY

Of course, even a failed technology is often the basis for further development. The lessons learned and the people trained by the endeavor creates the ability to do the next design. Engineers and programmers at Xerox's Palo Alto Research Center tried to invent a paperless document system and produced no profitable products. Apple took the ideas and the people and invented the Lisa computer, another market failure. Taking the best talents from that project and the lessons learned allowed the development of the Apple Macintosh. Copying the best features and strategies resulted in the Windows operating system, which is today's market leader and the de facto standard.

Understanding the Market

In his whole life, Vincent Van Gogh is said to have sold one painting, basically relying upon funds from his brother to buy bread and paint. But few modern creators have the same luxury (or are willing to live in such poverty). So our efforts must not only yield great creativity, they must trigger a flow of funds from the market economy that allow us to indulge our passion for design and creativity.

In art, there is an advantage to uniqueness, but in products and technology there is often a strong advantage to being the same as everyone else, thus sharing the costs of support services. Therefore, most technological marketing is either about becoming the market dominator or fitting your product to the market dominator. QWERTY is the market dominator. Kids in school are taught the keyboard. Anyone who has ever taken typing classes knows that keyboard. When you hire a temporary worker, they know that keyboard. It is hard to imagine any of the technically superior keyboards that have been developed ever gathering enough usage to justify investment in support and training.

Management of the approach to the market can be critical. Sony's Betamax and Apple's Macintosh are two technologies with a lot of lonely fans, frustrated as technologies they consider inferior dominate their marketplaces. It may be as simple as these two firms overestimating the premium they could charge in the market, a little too confident of their technical advantage. For example, while Betamax gave superior visual quality, most people were taking family films or converting various 8mm films to video to play through their older, lower quality televisions, places where Betamax's video fidelity gave little or no added benefit, so the customers simply would not pay the premium. On the other hand, while lacking visual fidelity, the VHS design had a robust simplicity that might be more tolerant of consumer errors as well as a length that could hold a whole movie. If first run movies had been made available more quickly to the video market, and if people's home televisions had larger and clearer screens, Betamax probably could have gotten away with the premium. If they had better understood their market position, they might have "given away" their technical advantage to customers and competed on equal price with VHS, obliterating that technology and funding the development and improvement of many video products.

Apple charged a similar premium price for the Macintosh because of its quality of graphics and ease of use. This was great for artists and teachers, but there were so many people who only needed word processing and spreadsheets, and who felt empowered, not frustrated, by the openness of the DOS-based systems that the volume went to the IBM compatible market. As hardware costs plummeted in a large (and growing), available DOS marketplace, Microsoft could afford to develop Windows to match many of the benefits of the Macintosh, and at lower cost per machine. Microsoft's market dominance now makes it easy to generate additional cash with various upgrades and new releases, cash that can fund new developments.

It is often dangerous to count on your own employees or the earliest adopters of technology to guide development of products for the masses. In the early 1950s at General Electric, management began to realize they had problems in the design of kitchen appliances for the consumers. For example, they noticed that to the well-educated electrical engineers they had hired to design electric ranges and cooking stoves, a superior design was one that most efficiently converted electricity to heat, which was not the concern highest in the consumer's mind. So they hired a chef to come in and teach the engineers to cook on those ranges. After this experience they began to make improvements to design that actually helped the homemaker. Of course, it never occurred to them to hire some housewives to be designers. And if you have ever owned one of those General Electric ranges from the late 1950s and early 1960s, it is obvious that the engineers never had to clean a stove, especially after several years of use.

This can all sound cynical and complaining, but success requires either incredible luck or careful attention to all the details, including how the product development and production will be funded. Thomas Edison was an inventor of this type. He set up an invention factory with various successful products funding the effort to develop new and better products. But he knew that without the ability for someone to make a successful business of his products, the products would never be made available. He not only supervised the invention of the incandescent light bulb, he worked diligently to provide everything an electric utility would need to operate—from generators to watt-meters, which allowed utilities to bill users for actual usage. It is easy to ignore such details or wait until some other inventor or entrepreneur finds the answer, but progress will move more quickly if the inventor accepts the need to invent a device that not only works for the customer but also for the marketplace that will deliver the product.

Pricing Free Services

What can really surprise people is the disconnect between price and benefit. Back when IBM sold mostly punch card sorters, their sorter came in two speeds, with the higher speed machine quite a bit more expensive. However, if you bought the lower speed machine, you could purchase a service upgrade to convert your machine to the higher speed for a price greater than the differential if you had originally bought the faster machine, but less than the cost of a second slow machine. As the story goes, if you purchased the upgrade, the service technician showed up with all kinds of tools and spare parts, then locked the customer out of the room while doing the long, tedious upgrade. Once the door was locked, the technician opened the toolbox, spread out the tools and spare parts, took out a thermos of coffee, a magazine, and maybe some snacks and read for a couple of hours. Then he put the magazine and coffee away, opened a panel and moved a drive belt from one drive wheel to another, ran a test on the machine speed, and invited the customer in for a demonstration. Some would complain that it was unfair, or even immoral, to sell a $25 adjustment for several thousand dollars, but the added function was certainly worth the price to the customer.

This customer value per cost is the main issue in technological success. The majority of telephone switches operated by the local telephone companies in the United States have the built-in capacity for services such as three-way calling, caller ID, speed dialing, and so on. In fact you cannot buy a switch today without these services. The added cost of providing these services to customers is basically zero. Yet the phone company is able to charge $3-$5 per month for each of these services. As long as this market lasts, the most valuable resource of a telephone company is gullible customers with no alternatives. This is why the road to corporate success in America's telephone systems today is to get a lot more of these gullible customers, thus leading to buying the other regional telephone companies as the fastest route to greater income.

This may seem unfair, but if these companies are legally able and willing to use that cash flow to accelerate the design evolution of the global telecommunication systems, it is a great process.

This high cost for free stuff also applies to software. Once a software package is written, the cost for each additional copy delivered can be as low as zero for downloaded software or $3 for a CD version. The ability to price such free goods in such a way as to fund the further development of products you are interested in is the real name of the game in managing technology.

CONCLUSIONS

So what is a designer to do in the current global explosion of health-related knowledge and technology? One option is to just relax and enjoy the ride. But for those who want to be players, it is important to become more broadly aware of the business, strategy, technology, and political issues relevant to the field and, more importantly, to develop relationships and collaborations that allow you to mobilize conversations that are capable of having a relevant AHA. Who do you need to know? What projects do you need to work on to be ready to develop worthwhile products?

The basic trick is humility—to recognize that you really do not understand the whole situation and that working alone you probably never will understand it well enough to make all the decisions. It also seems important to recognize that you might not be equipped by background, experience, and values to have AHAs about your technology that are relevant to the needs of the consumer whose money you want to pay your expenses while you play with the next generation of the technology.

Designing successful technologies takes both focused work on key technical issues and broad understanding of the complex realities of the users, the distributors, the producers, and all others involved in the network of activities to deliver health to people. The broad understanding of issues generally requires a creative collaborative interaction among those who know different parts of "the elephant." Such interaction requires the sharing of goals, strategies, and beliefs among the collaborators to develop a fuzzy mess of understanding of the complex dynamics of the problem situation. Such interaction can benefit from techniques developed by other designers, such as costed function analysis, decision criteria matrix, creative problem solving, brainstorming, and various team-building activities. Even covert usage of these guiding principles by participants in the collaboration can accelerate the synergy and co-creativity of collaborations, thus accelerating the design evolution, bringing more effective and efficient technologies into use sooner. The techniques and concepts are available, for those who have the will to make it happen.

NOTES

[1] Petroski, H., *Design Paradigms* (New York: Cambridge University Press, 1994).

[2] Barlow, C. M., "Deliberate Insight in Team Creativity," *Journal of Creative Behavior*, 34(2), 2000, 101–117.

[3] Koestler, A., *Janus* (New York: Random House, 1978).

[4] Simon, H., "The Proverbs of Administration," *Public Administration Review*, 6, 1946, 53–67.

[5] Nonaka, I., and H. Takeuchi, *The Knowledge Creating Company* (New York: Oxford University Press, 1995).

[6] Miles, L. D., *Techniques of Value Engineering and Analysis* (2nd ed.) (New York: McGraw-Hill, 1971).

[7] Mudge, A. E., *Value Engineering* (New York: McGraw-Hill, 1971).

[8] Fowler, T. C., *Value Analysis in Design* (New York: Van Nostrand Reinhold, 1990).

[9] Snodgrass, T. J., and M. Kasi, *Function Analysis: The Stepping Stones to Good Value* (Madison: University of Wisconsin Press, 1986).

Chapter 6

Strategic Planning in Healthcare Organizations: The Role of Health Technology Assessment

Americo Cicchetti

INTRODUCTION

The main aim of this chapter is to define the possible role that principles and tools of Health Technology Assessment (HTA) can play in the hospital's strategic planning process. A few large hospitals around the world are testing the use of HTA for strategic decision making and, in particular, for the adoption of new technologies and the establishment of new services. This chapter discusses some theoretical issues and reports on the experience of a large teaching hospital in Italy during its implementation of HTA.

Strategic planning is crucial in the management of healthcare organizations, even when the characteristics of the healthcare systems vary. Public hospital trusts (in Italy and in other countries), as well as private non-profit and for-profit hospitals, are called to continuously improve their managerial processes, with particular attention on the efficacy of the strategic planning models applied.

One of the well-recognized pitfalls of the strategic planning process approach is related to the existing dualism between "formulation" and "implementation" phases. Internal organizational conditions, emerging strategies, and changes in external environment typically place the implementation phase in jeopardy. This problem seems to be harder to solve in the case of hospitals.

In healthcare organizations, the clinical autonomy of physicians, in conjunction with their direct responsibility for patients, makes it difficult to apply formal planning and budgeting processes. Thus, a hospital is viewed as a loosely coupled system. Healthcare activities and clinical processes are difficult to predict in terms of volumes and quality. Under these conditions, strategies tend to emerge from the bottom and implementation of deliberated strategies by the top management team become particularly complex.

Starting from this position, this chapter suggests how the HTA framework might provide solutions to the problem of effective strategic planning processes in healthcare organizations.

BACKGROUND

For the last 15 years, European countries have been involved in a large reform program of their healthcare systems. The first "movers" of these reforms were pressure for cost containment and the need to rationalize the use of resources. An aging population, the increasing demand for services, and technological innovation in medicine represent the main factors in the increasing gap between needs and resources available for health care. Many countries, before experimenting with more critical decisions (rationing and prioritization), proposed a different way to distribute use resource. The solution is based on enhancing the effectiveness and efficiency of clinical and administrative processes in hospitals and healthcare organizations. This objective was pursued by increasing the level of autonomy of healthcare organizations with respect to national formal planning processes (so called "managerial revolution"), and experimenting with a quasi-markets solution [1].

More recently, some European countries (the United Kingdom and Italy, for example) voted legislation that limited the impact of market mechanisms in healthcare systems. Nevertheless, countries all over Europe are stressing the relevance of managerial principles and tools to improve the effectiveness and efficiency of their healthcare systems.

Recent innovations in the statutes of the Italian National Health Service have enlarged the autonomy of healthcare organizations (Legislative Decree No. 229/1999), evoking a proportional recognition of the criticality of strategic planning process in the business of government. The definition of the mission and the objectives, the selection of strategic options [2, 3], the formulation of strategies, their implementation, and their evaluation all represent the fundamental steps of this process (see Figure 6.1).

The effectiveness of the strategic planning process can be measured by its ability to produce maximum value for the different stakeholders in the health system, namely, the patients, the statutes from which the institution derives part of its objectives, and the institution itself. These components compose the organizational unity.

The strategic planning process has particular connotations in health organizations.

Figure 6.1
Strategic Planning Process in Healthcare Organizations

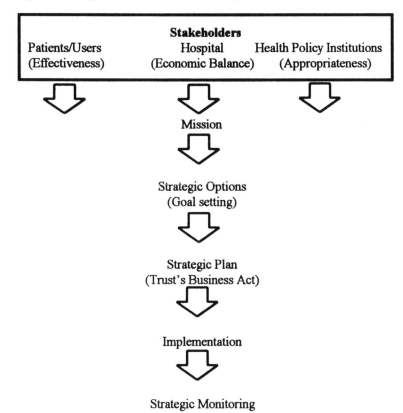

The Importance of Institutional Rules and the Limitation of "Strategic Space" [4]

Healthcare organizations operate in an environment contemporarily responding to "technical" and "institutional" rules [5].

Recent reforms of healthcare systems in European countries have minimized the dominance of "institutional" rules (such as legislation or legitimization of a hospital in the social and political environment) toward more emphasis on, and influence of, managerial decisions—where technical rules such as efficiency, effectiveness, and efficacy define the new framework for managerial choices [6].

In Italy, similar to other European countries, the "managerial revolution" of the early 1990s (started with Leg. Decree 502/1992) suggests a new institutional framework for healthcare management.

The healthcare organization, besides having its own mission, has a function to meet the objectives defined by the Italian National Health Service [7]. Such a situation limits the so called "strategic space" of the heads of Italian hospitals [8, 9], thus reducing their discretionary power. The hospitals' strategic plan (PSA) [10] represents the final part of a wider planning process that involves central organs (National Health Plan), regional authorities (Regional Health Plan), and local health authorities (Local Operational Plan, Art. 2, Leg. Decree No. 229/1999).

Hospitals as Knowledge-Based Organizations

Healthcare organizations, namely hospitals, belong to those fields that have been defined as *science (or knowledge) based* [11]. Success in such sectors seems to be strictly related to the managerial ability to run, develop, promote, and recombine core competencies [12] in first-rate healthcare processes. In hospitals, the strategic planning process cannot ignore accumulated knowledge as a primary source of inspiration for strategic choices [13].

The "Weakness of Ties" in Hospitals

The worker's professional autonomy designates the healthcare organization as a "weakly coupled system" [14, 15]. The effectiveness of formal planning systems is limited in their traditional form, creating difficulties in the implementation of managerial strategic choices because of an organizational texture characterized by a system of values and incentives extremely difficult to manage [16].

These considerations suggest that the supply of the traditional tools supporting the process of strategic planning are insufficient to successfully face the issues deriving from the characteristics of the health organizations discussed above. The considerations that follow, starting from the evaluation of the above-said characteristics, provide a few guidelines to promote the effectiveness of the strategic planning process in healthcare organizations:

- Pointing out the possible tools to reduce the dichotomy between formulation and strategic implementation, underlining, at the same time, how critical it is to select strategic planning that reduces this dichotomy;
- Offering a method that contributes to a more effective process of selecting the options fostering, *ex-ante*, the implementation by the organizational "texture."

THE SELECTION OF STRATEGIC OPTIONS

As in many other sectors, the effectiveness of formulating strategies in health care involves bringing together the formulation-implementation effort [17, 18]. Different aspects within the healthcare sector make such recomposition particularly difficult to establish:

- The "turbulence" of the statutes makes particularly aleatory the implementation of decided plans, which are incoherent and weak as a result of changes in the context.
- The autonomy and the professional orientations of physicians [19] create the emergence of "strategies from below," often creating conflicts between orientations of managers and individual goals (professional and/or scientific goals). The different values that characterize clinicians and managers, the different perception of institutional realities, and often the lack of a systemic and strategic vision shared within the hospital make rather aleatory the realization of strategic plans proposed by management.
- Surpassing institutional and social obligations create the inability to exert pressure in certain areas of management (for example, human resources).

In healthcare institutions an efficient strategic planning process—able to timely define, consistently implement its options, and encourage the achievement of the mission and the production of value for all the *stakeholders*—implies the necessity to identify tools that are able to select the "options" in a more consistent way in comparison with the implementation area.

Therefore, it is not advisable to forgo any "planning" effort but to identify tools that are capable of screening what can be done with different strategic options (the so-called "sieve of the feasibility"), formalizing, in the strategic planning process, only those contents that will find a "munificent" environment of application in the organization [20].

The previous considerations are advanced to underline the criticality of selection of strategic options and, therefore, of the content of fulfilling strategic plans. In a clear and unequivocal way, previous studies have defined the survey of options available to managers of healthcare organizations, such as:

- The rationalization of resource use;
- The growth of productivity of infrastructures and other key resources;
- The activation of a process of continuous quality improvement, accumulating and exploiting sources of competitive advantage; and
- The redefinition of the mix of strategic services and typologies of services to optimize the allocation of the resources.

While the first two options aim to keep the organizational system alive, helping to achieve the economic balance in the short-middle range, projects concerning the last two options concern the organization over a longer time period. The scheme in Figure 6.2 underlines this dualism but

Figure 6.2
Strategic Options in Healthcare Organizations

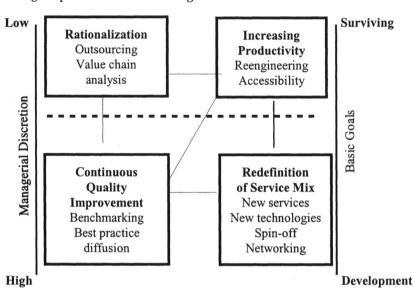

Source: Adapted by the author from Ginter, Swayne, and Duncan, 1997 [2].

also shows the close interactions among strategic plans implemented in different areas.

The first category of strategic options includes the revision of acquisition of key resources, such as pharmaceutical, prosthetic, and the outsourcing processes of some activities in order to contain costs and to focus on clinical core services. The second option, for instance, can be carried out by simplifying healthcare or administrative processes through business process reengineering programs.

In the second area, the projects of continuous quality improvement are often inspired by institutional requirements (e.g., accreditation processes) and are more easily shared by different professional members. The exception occurs when problems arise relating to lack of competencies, time, and decision-making processes.

The redefinition of the mix of healthcare services also involves other issues. It imposes discretionary choices of resource allocation (current and capital expenditures) that should be based on a managerial rationality built through the recognition of the resources, the internal competencies, and through the analysis of the task environment. Apart from the degree of competence of heads of institutions, every discretionary choice of a "nonphysician" manager in the field of medicine causes reactions and obstacles in the implementation within the organization and, particularly, among professionals. The arising conflicts, reactions, and inactivities aimed to slow down the innovation process in the organization can be overcome with a little effort.

THE ROLE OF THE HEALTH TECHNOLOGY ASSESSMENT IN THE SELECTION OF STRATEGIC OPTIONS

The discretionary power that characterizes the redefinition of the mix of services provides tools that ensure the strategic coherence of the different changes already started and, at the same time, their approval both by the organization and the professional members.

Some innovative experiences in the United States, the Netherlands, Canada, and Italy [21] underline the emergence of a management pattern of innovation in the medical field that seems to promise to overcome issues of integration between the phases of formulation and implementation of discretionary strategic options.

This pattern uses methodologies developed within the multidisciplinary scientific field known as HTA [22]. The methodologies of HTA ensure a multidisciplinary evaluation of health technologies such as medical devices, drugs, organizational procedures, and diagnostic and therapeutic courses [23].

The "assessment of technologies" (synthesis of an evaluation of appropriateness, efficiency, effectiveness, and quality) requires multidisciplinary competencies in the different clinical areas of epidemiology, biostatistics, economy, and management. These competencies are mainly used to support policymaking so that the scientific subject is suitable for evaluation by a nontechnical policymaker [24]. Recently, these competencies have been tested to support strategic decision making at the hospital level [25, 26].

Such methodologies are essential for a comparative and scientifically strong evaluation of the different choices in the innovation of services (or of technologies) deriving from clinicians (generally from chief of departments), and in helping to redefine the mix of services supported by the structure.

The goal is to create within the hospital a competitive arena of innovative ideas that in some respect help to get sponsorship from management and their business strategic plans (intended as tools of realization of strategic options). Within this model, management should play a role of *sponsor* of the creativity of clinicians, spurring them to provide new services in reply to outstanding needs or rising technologies.

Specifically assigned units can be organized to carry out tasks of advising clinicians, supporting them with economic and financial evaluations (business planning) of the innovation process.

With top management's direction, such units define a few guidelines for the formulation of proposals to support in different phases. The guidelines tend to provide a pre-filter of innovations, since physicians are asked to supply a plan with:

- A review of available scientific evidence to support the appropriateness of the new service or the new suggested technology in conformity with the approach of *evidence-based medicine* [27].
- The factors that determine the coherence of the proposed service with underlying strategic guidelines and with infrastructural and organizational linkages (e.g., work force and its reorganization).
- An evaluation of the economic sustainability of the project. Such sustainability should be supported with an adequate *business plan* that underlines costs and differential proceeds both current and future (new technologies, new spaces).
- An inquiry of the present and potential areas of application for the new service and the new technologies.
- The discussion of ethical issues.

This first phase, which actually develops without solution of continuity and therefore not necessarily in concomitance with the drawing up of the long-term strategic plan, allows management to have an outline of appropriate options of financing by the regional Health Service (or of other payor) and of the efficiency and effectiveness of the system. These pre-filtered options redefine managerial decision making that has to assess the coherence and both the economic-financial and the strategic organizational feasibility.

In the overall management of health institutions, the guidelines described above seem to ensure:

- A specific orientation of the organization to innovation in clinical research and in organizational and healthcare processes. This is due to the participation and responsibility of the professionals.
- A continuous improvement of appropriateness of services; each new service (or technology) is previously examined and evaluated.
- A new way of communication between top management and clinicians on a cultural and linguistic level that is appropriate to the scientific culture of physicians.
- The possibility to strengthen the leadership of managers who observe the rules of evidence-based strategic management.
- The chance to strengthen "centers of excellence" in hospitals [28], since the investments seem to reward those who are at the height of science, hence combining the ability to foster knowledge-creation processes, with the ability of implementing this knowledge in new organizational routines.

Table 6.1
Policlinico A. Gemelli and Columbus Hospital, Rome (1999 Fact Sheet)

Acute ordinary beds	1,915
Day hospital beds	213
Ordinary discharges	58,951
Number of day cases	71,096
Number of outpatients	1,383,355
Number of medical doctors	736
Other personnel	3,750
Budget	310 million euros

THE HEALTH TECHNOLOGY ASSESSMENT UNIT (HTA-U) AT A. GEMELLI TEACHING HOSPITAL

Policlinico Agostino Gemelli is the teaching hospital of the School of Medicine of the Catholic University of Rome (UCSC). Under this definition it is considered a complex and integrated healthcare delivery system providing acute hospital care (inpatient and outpatient), hospice care, and home care.

Acute care is ensured by four different hospitals: Policlinico A. Gemelli (1,615 acute beds), Columbus Hospital (300 acute beds) in UCSC Campus in Rome; Celano Hospital (200 acute beds) (Abruzzo region), Research Hospital of Campobasso (about 400 acute beds under construction) (Molise Region). These sites provide day-hospital/day-surgery acute care and a wide range of outpatient services (see Table 6.1).

Hospice care for the elderly is provided in two different settings: in the UCSC campus in Rome (90 beds) and in Fontecchio (Abruzzo Region—200 beds).

In order to support the top management team in the decision-making process, the Health Technology Assessment Unit (HTAU) was established in 2000. The top management team felt the need to create a new multidisciplinary unit at the corporate level to monitor, assess, and promote the use of new technologies throughout the system. HTAU was provided with a complex set of responsibilities: management of quality improvement projects, management of benchmarking projects, and assessment of existing medical technologies and new investments.

By performing this assessment the HTAU is playing a critical role in the strategic planning process. It is a collector of needs (clinical, organizational, and managerial) and is responsible for summarizing these

Table 6.2
Competencies and Affiliations for HTA-U

Competencies	Affiliations
Epidemiologists, Biostatisticians, Economists	University–Institute of Hygiene and Public Health
Clinical Management	Medical Directorate
Accounting and Financial Control	Financial Control and Planning Unit
Engineers	Technical Support Services Team
Clinical Competencies	University–Clinical Institutes

needs and producing information for the development of a technology investment plan, which is a critical part of the three-year strategic plan.

HTAU is operating as a staff consultant group of the Medical Directorate, relying on competencies and information from other hospital or university departments (see Table 6.2).

The process of HTAU decision making was designed with the objective of assessing technologies so that the organization may:

- Assess the improvement in the efficiency and effectiveness of clinical processes that rely on the new technology;
- Assess the appropriateness of services provided within the new technology;
- Assess the coherence of the new services produced with the new technology, within the framework of the hospital's strategic plan, and
- Assess the internal coherence of different technological investments designed to penetrate new healthcare markets.

The HTAU activity is based on a typical Health Technology Assessment approach, which considers all information to be useful in the formulation of the hospital's technology investment plan. This plan is based on evidence, according to the evidence-based medicine framework.

The activity of the HTAU is also based on continuous exchange of information and advice with clinical departments. Early findings from our studies show how meta-analysis and other tools providing scientific evidence for decision-making processes make the top management's team investment and strategic plans more likely to be accepted by department chiefs.

Discussions about new investments and service restructuring, performed on a scientific base, are more likely to produce rational solutions coherent with strategic long range planning.

In the University Hospital Agostino Gemelli, the HTA process is following these steps:

23. Strategic planning—Budget for investment (Proposal) (September Y_n);
24. Elaboration and diffusion of Guidelines for Technology Needs Assessment (July–September Y_n);
25. Technology needs assessment (hospital departments) (September–November Y_n);
26. HTA-team evaluation process (November–December Y_n);
27. Investment plan (December Y_n);
28. Budget for investment: Adoption (January Y_{n+1}).

CONCLUSION

The methodological approach described some of the difficulties of applying strategic planning process in healthcare organizations. In the first place, it seems to abide by the institutional rules that require healthcare organizations to consider objectives of low costs, quality, and the strengthening of the reputation of the organization vis-à-vis the regional healthcare market regulators and the patients.

Secondly, the approach focuses on the accumulated scientific knowledge in the hospital, thus exploiting its potential. The redefinition of the mix of services and, more generally, the selection of strategic options is applied by giving an important role to the activities emerging from the hospital routine. Such an approach has inherent conflicts, which characterize a process of strategic planning in which there is a distinction between the formulation of strategy by the elite and activities of the implementation phase.

The arguments presented in this chapter suggest that the reduction of the dichotomy formulation-implementation in healthcare organizations can be attenuated by adopting an approach that is contemporarily *knowledge based* and *evidence based*. Principles and tools elaborated in the multidisciplinary setting of HTA seem to be useful in promoting a strategic management process that is rooted in the evidence- and knowledge-based approach.

On the one hand, what has been said stresses the wideness of the strategic space available to heads of the present institutional set-up of the Italian NHS (similarly to many other UE countries). On the other hand, it suggests new responsibilities for managers and clinicians.

As far as the top management team is concerned, the choice of a new managerial style is a tool that utilizes evidence in a key role within the strategic decision strategic process. This style uses methodologies of business administration developed in the field of strategic management.

As for clinicians, it seems necessary to be aware of the responsibilities deriving from their managerial role in modern healthcare organizations. This imposes a change that may be accomplished both through training and awareness by clinicians in order to spread a systemic and strategic vision.

NOTES

[1] Saltman, R. B., and C. Van Otter, *Implementing Planned Markets in Health Care* (London: Open University Press, 1995).

[2] Ginter P. M., L. M. Swayne, and J. W. Duncan, *Strategic Management of Healthcare Organizations* (Cambridge: Blackwell Publishers, 1997).

[3] Achard, P. O., *Economia E Organizzazione Delle Imprese Sanitarie* (Milano: Franco Angeli, 1999).

[4] This expression is used to indicate the scope of autonomy granted to hospitals' top management team in the strategic planning process.

[5] Scott, W. R., and J. Meyer, *Organizational Environments: Ritual and Rationality* (Beverly Hills, CA: Sage Publications, 1983).

[6] Ferlie, E., L. Ashburner, L. Fitzgerald, and A. Pettigrew, *The New Public Management in Action* (Oxford: Oxford University Press, 1996).

[7] Borgonovi, E., "Il Controllo Economico Nelle Aziende Con Processi Ad Elevata Autonomia Professionale," in Borgonovi, E. (Ed.), *Il Controllo Economico Nelle Aziende Sanitarie* (Milano: Egea, 1990).

[8] Rebora, G., and M. Meneguzzo, *Strategia delle Amministrazioni Pubbliche* (Torino: UTET, 1990).

[9] Fontana, F., and G. Lorenzoni in Fontana, F., and G. Lorenzoni (Eds.), *L'architettura Strategica Delle Aziende Ospedaliere: Una Analisi Empirica* (Milano: Franco Angeli, 2000).

[10] In the present set-up of healthcare statutes the PSA is an integral part of the business act of private law and an essential tool for elaborating the long-term budget in public and accredited hospitals (Leg. Ve Decree n. 229/1999).

[11] Foss, N. J., "Knowledge-Based Approaches to The Theory of The Firm: Some Critical Comments," *Organization Science*, 7(5), 1996, 470–476.

[12] Prahalad, C., and G. Hamel, "The Core Competence of the Corporation," *Harvard Business Review*, May–June 1990, 79–89.

[13] Cicchetti, A., and G. Lorenzoni, "L'architettura Strategica Delle Aziende Sanitarie: Una Prospettiva Basata Sulle Conoscenze," in Fontana, F. and G. Lorenzoni (Eds.), *L'architettura Strategica Delle Aziende Sanitarie: Una Analisi Empirica* (Milano: Franco Angeli, 2000).

[14] Weick, K. E., "Educational Organizations as Loosely Coupled Systems," *Administrative Science Quarterly*, 22, March 1976, 1–19.

[15] Covaleski, M. A., and M. W. Dirsmith, "Budgeting as a Means for Control and Loose Coupling," *Accounting, Organizations and Society*, 88(4), 1983, 323–240.

[16] Friedson, E., *Professional Dominance: the Social Structure of Medical Care* (New York: Atherton Press, 1970).

[17] Fontana, F., *Il Sistema Organizzativo Aziendale* (Milano: Franco Angeli, 1997).

[18] Mintzberg, H., "The Rise and Fall of Strategic Planning," *Harvard Business Review*, January–February 1994.

[19] Guerra, G., *Psicologia dell'ospedale: Analisi Organizzativa e Processi di Cambiamento* (Roma: NIS, 1992).

[20] Achard, P. O., A. Cicchetti, and S. Profili, "La Formazione Delle Strategie Nelle Aziende Sanitarie," in Fontana, F., and G. Lorenzoni (eds.), *L'architettura Strategica Delle Aziende Ospedaliere: Una Analisi Empirica* (Milano: Franco Angeli, 2000).

[21] In 2000, the A. Gemelli University Hospital (Rome) started a Technology Assessment Unit that applies some of the solutions shown here. Such experiences are also being conducted at the Consortium of the University Hospitals at McGill University (Montreal), the Baylor Health System (Dallas, TX), and the University Hospital of Amsterdam.

[22] Institute of Medicine, *Assessing Medical Technology* (Washington, DC: National Academy Press, 1985).

[23] Fuchs, V. R., *The Future of Health Policy* (Cambridge, MA: Harvard University Press, 1993).

[24] Battista, R. N., "Innovation and Diffusion of Health-Related Technologies: A Conceptual Framework," *International Journal of Technology Assessment in Health Care*, 5(2), 1989, 227–248.

[25] Luce, B. R., and R. E. Brown, "The Use of Technology Assessment by Hospitals, Health Maintenance Organizations, and Third-Party Payers in the United States," *International Journal of Technology Assessment in Health Care*, 11(1), 1995, 79–92.

[26] Cicchetti, A., G. C. Vanini, C. Catananti, A. Cicchetti, and M. Marchetti, "The Role of Health Technology Assessment in the Hospital Management: The HTA Team in a Large Teaching Hospital" (paper presented at the Annual Meeting of the International Society of Technology Assessment in Health Care [ISTAHC], Edinburgh, June 1998).

[27] Sackett, D., "Evidence-Based Medicine," *Lancet*, 346(8983), 1995, 1171.

[28] Grandi, A., and G. Lorenzoni, "Center of Excellence in Healthcare Organizations," working Paper, Università degli Studi di Bologna, Department of Management, 1999.

Chapter 7

Diagnostic and Information Technology for Laboratories in an Integrated Delivery System

Craig A. Lehmann and John Fitzgibbon

INTRODUCTION

Healthcare facilities in all parts of the world have tried to address the ever-changing healthcare system. In the United States the creation of a community-based integrated delivery system appears to be the strategy of choice among most healthcare facilities [1]. The design and intricacy of these systems vary among healthcare facilities. For example, some just have shared services (i.e., laboratory and/or radiology services), while others are far more multifaceted (i.e., the integration of healthcare services that provides a continuum of services from the tertiary care hospital to the patient's home). Such community-based integrated delivery systems can eliminate redundancy in their services and achieve economies of scale by "channeling" patients to the appropriate facility to deliver treatment in the most cost-effective way. Hospitals can be owned by one entity, for-profit corporation or not-for-profit entity, or have separate ownership but form the network to achieve economies and negotiate managed-care contracts for the network.

The integration of laboratory services with a regional core laboratory seems to have the greatest impact on improving efficiency and decreasing costs [2]. In this scenario the core laboratory is usually placed at a tertiary care and/or teaching hospital where the testing is more sophisticated and personnel is at a higher level (i.e., Ph.D.). The remaining facilities have full service laboratories, rapid-response laboratories or STAT laboratories. On rare occasions, the regional laboratory is a free-standing structure. The regional core laboratory can have a variety of functions: it can perform the majority of all testing for the region, or it can be the centralized testing for outreach, low-volume esoteric testing, or other testing where turnaround time is not critical.

Some community-based integrated systems have elected to distribute laboratory testing to hospitals based upon their comparative advantage. For example, if one hospital has a specialty in virology and performs relatively high volumes of testing, it should be considered the desirable site for that area of testing.

Some of the earlier systems implemented only STAT capabilities at all hospital laboratories, other than the one that housed the core laboratory. This strategy was short lived, as most hospitals found that physicians needed many of the routine tests, and their absence had a negative impact on patient length of stay in the hospital. Because of this and other reasons, most hospital laboratories have fully automated rapid response laboratories that process tests in "real time." To accomplish this goal, automated instrumentation for chemistry, immunology, hematology, coagulation, and urinalysis should be available at each facility and located in one open room. This streamlines workflow, improves turnaround time, enhances communication among staff, and maximizes the advantages of cross-training. Samples from all areas of the hospital should be sent to central accessioning for processing. It is best when these samples are sent via pneumatic tubes, thereby helping the lab meet turnaround time requirements.

With this configuration, the additional laboratory space or personnel needed to process all of these highly automated tests on site is minimal when compared to a STAT-only model. Current instrumentation, with bar code readers, high throughput, direct tube sampling, and other labor-saving features minimize labor. As such, staffing required to process additional samples or perform more tests, (i.e., a Chem 20 profile versus the Chem 7 STAT panel) are comparable. The additional instrumentation costs are also minimal. This obviates the need to pack samples and move them to a central off-site location. Samples collected from physicians' offices, physicians' office laboratories, nursing homes, or clinics are processed at the designated regional laboratory.

INTEGRATED DELIVERY SYSTEMS

Laboratories in a community-based integrated system are currently attempting to standardize their technology as well as their information systems. This change will reduce costs through sharing of reagents and supplies. As patients move through the system, their laboratory reference ranges will remain the same, therefore allowing physicians to compare previous data and better monitor changes in test results. While this might have been difficult to do a few years ago, it can be done today. This is primarily due to the recent introduction of technology with varying throughputs and the breadth of technology by a single vendor [3]. A large hospital can utilize a similar instrument with the same methodologies as a smaller hospital.

While the laboratory and other strategies vary among community-based integrated systems, all have attempted to reduce a patient's hospital length of stay. Under the U.S. reimbursement system, Diagnostic Related Groups (DRGs), which reduce the patient's length of stay, provide economic gains. This reduction of patient stay has significantly decreased the number of hospital beds in the United States. Another outcome of this reimbursement policy has been to send patients home earlier, even though many still require the attention of healthcare providers (e.g., registered nurses). This has created some concerns for many healthcare payors (i.e., private insurance and government healthcare payors), as they are realizing increased costs in home health care.

In addition to the growing number of patients needing health services after their hospital stay, the United States is faced with a growing population of aged citizens (65 years or older). The projections are that there will be more than 69 million individuals over 65 years of age by the year 2030. Presently in the United States, when an individual reaches the age of 65 he or she is entitled to health insurance by the government (Medicare). The U.S. government is concerned that the numbers and long-term chronic ailments of this aged population will place an economic strain on the healthcare system.

In 1997, 3.5 million Medicare enrollees received home health services—an increase of about 100 percent since 1990. The 1999 cost for home health care reached $36 billion and is expected to grow substantially [4]. Most of this growth is due to a patient's decreased length of hospital stay. However, the greater growth in home health will not be seen until the year 2013 when the "Baby Boomers" are first predicted to enter the Medicare system.

Many health care agencies today realize the key to cost containment is better management of the patient. Better management not only improves the patient's well being, it reduces the number of encounters that the patient has with emergency departments, hospital admissions, and possibly visits to the physician's office. There are three key elements in providing economical patient management outside the hospital: self-testing, connectivity, and telemedicine. Telemedicine will play a vital role in providing home health care, especially now that real-time visualization of the patient can occur.

TELEMEDICINE TECHNOLOGY

The introduction of telemedicine technology that allows visualization of both the practitioner and patient as well as the collection of clinical data is a major breakthrough for this market. For example, the technology offered by HomMed Sentry collects the patient's heart rate, blood pressure, O_2 saturation, weight, and temperature. In addition, some of the technology will have ports, which enable patients to connect a spirometer and POCT technology (e.g., glucose monitor).

Over the same time period there has been an increase in the number of approved point-of-care testing methods for self-testing, which will allow patients to send their self-test results via their vital sign technology. Self-testing and telemedicine will provide needed economical means for managing patients in a community-based healthcare system (ambulatory care). One of the largest costs of providing health care to homebound patients is labor. Sending a healthcare provider to a patient's residence, either to visit the patient or collect a laboratory sample, is very expensive. Telemedicine should help decrease overall costs of labor, since vendors have demonstrated that a home healthcare nurse can see more than double the number of patients when using telemedicine. The other element that is helping to decrease costs of the homebound patient is "patient management." Research has demonstrated that management of homebound patients not only expedites recovery but decreases the patient's encounters with emergency departments, hospitals, and/or physicians' offices.

In the future, the management of the patient in a community-based healthcare system, especially when home health care is a component, will rely heavily on information systems. The connectivity will be somewhat complex. However, this connectivity will be a necessary component if the community-based healthcare system is going to provide an efficient and economical system.

The process of connecting hospital clinical laboratories in a community-based healthcare system has been very slow even without home health care. This has been because many hospital laboratories have different laboratory information systems (LIS) and the replacement of these systems to create one common LIS would be costly. This would be compounded even further if the community-based system tried to integrate home healthcare data into their LIS system. However, just recently some LIS vendors have offered application service provisioning as a solution. An application service provider (ASP) deploys, hosts, and manages software applications, which in return could reduce the costs of standardizing laboratory information systems. Under the ASP model there is the potential to reduce costs by 30 to 60 percent. ASPs provide the infrastructure and support services without hardware costs. A full service ASP offers continuous access to their latest technology. They take on full responsibility for maintaining the information technology. This in turn allows hospitals to spend less on information technology personnel and spend more on other operations.

It is obvious that the next few years will truly change the way we deliver health care. Economics will continue to drive the change, while diagnostic and information technology will provide the tools to make it happen.

NOTES

[1] Schumm C., W. H. Thurstoon, and R. I. Weiss, "Integrated Laboratory Networks: Ideas That Work," *Medical Laboratory Observer*, 31(2), 1999, 18–25.

[2] Salhany R., "Re-engineering to the Core Lab Concept," *Advanced Administration Laboratory*, 10(4), 1998, 19–22.

[3] Lehmann C. A., and A. M. Leiken, "The Consolidation Chase: A Key to Improving Efficiency," *Advanced Administration Laboratory*, 4(8), 1995, 36–42.

[4] www.nach.org/consumer/hcstats.html, home care statistics, November 2000.

Chapter 8

Using Diagnostic Workshops to Achieve Excellence in the NHS

Alex Appleby and Maxine Conner

INTRODUCTION

The main aim of this chapter is to report initial findings of a collaborative venture between the Northern and Yorkshire Learning Alliance NHS and the Newcastle Business School's Center for Business Excellence at the University of Northumbria. The focus of the collaboration is to increase awareness and gain wider acceptance for the principles of "excellence" in the NHS (National Health Service). The chapter is written in five sections. First is a short background review that examines the current drivers for health care in the United Kingdom. The NHS Plan, Department of Health [1], sets out a radical vision with a 10-year implementation time frame. At the heart of the plan are the concepts of excellence embodied within the European Foundation for Quality Management (EFQM) Excellence Model [2]. The second section describes the collaboration and explains how the project team introduces NHS organizations to the principles of excellence by using a diagnostic benchmarking tool. It discusses the methodology used in the pilot phase of the work and examines the links with the EFQM model. The third section gives details of those NHS organizations that have been involved so far and reports some outcomes from the workshop activities. The next section gives insight into views obtained during post-workshop interviews with NHS staff. The chapter concludes with a summary of the overall benefits of the diagnostic workshop and outlines future work planned by the partnership.

BACKGROUND AND REVIEW OF LITERATURE

The NHS Framework for Quality, Department of Health [3] emphasizes the importance of creating an environment in which "excellence" can flourish. It places clear responsibilities on chief executives, trust boards, and individuals to base practice on sound research evidence and to monitor the outcomes of care through audit activity. Central to quality strategy is the Clinical Governance Framework, which incorporates clinical risk management, accountability of the organization and individuals, and performance management. It stresses the need to examine processes to assure quality and value for money.

Guidance produced by the NHS Executive in 1999 [4] accentuates the need for a human resources strategy focusing on developing leadership, people management, resource sharing, and partnership working, and stresses the quality of service delivery. This, together with the focus upon the "patient journey" or process of care delivery identified in the NHS Plan, DOH 2000 [1] clearly illustrates the overall focus of the areas of excellence identified within the EFQM Excellence Model. This approach clearly identifies that improved business "results" are achieved through successful management and improvement of "enablers." The plan builds upon earlier policy documents stressing that service must satisfy its customers with ever-improving standards of care and must offer its staff a positive work experience.

COLLABORATION AND METHODOLOGY

The Northern and Yorkshire Learning Alliance (NYLA), set up in 1999, operates as part of the NHS Learning Network (http://www.nyx. org.uk). The organization operates in a "virtual" manner, providing service improvement support to NHS teams that are working to modernize their services. The organization has a small core team (10 staff members) who provide support to organizations in a geographic area covering 10,000 square miles. NYLA, developed with government funding from the Department of Health, aims to develop NHS capacity for learning and service improvement. NYLA has three core processes:

• Service improvement project development and support process
• Sharing practice process
• Training and development process

The other partner in this collaboration is the Center for Business Excellence (CfBE; http://be.unn.ac.uk) with a small research team of seven, which is part of the Newcastle Business School at the University of

Northumbria. The center, formed in 1999, resulted from the successful completion of a three-year research project that looked at the competitiveness of manufacturing and service industries in the northeast region of the United Kingdom [5–7]. The center was chosen by NYLA as a partner because of its experience in the development of diagnostic assessment tools and experience in working with other organizations in their pursuit of excellence.

The partnership between NYLA and CfBE was formed during 2000. Its purpose is to assist NHS managers and clinicians to assess their practices and performance against the standards of "business excellence" and to plan and implement improvements. Early signs indicate that it is already developing into a powerful learning partnership.

The first stage of the new partnership's work has focused on the development of a healthcare diagnostic benchmarking tool and its deployment through a series of pilot workshops in NHS Trust organizations. At this time (and for the purpose of this chapter) it is likely that the completed version of the tool will be called "PROBE for Health Care." The ultimate aim of the partnership is to help NHS organizations identify strengths and areas for improvements within their service provision. Using such a tool in this way can also assist NHS organizations in their understanding of the principles of the (EFQM) Excellence Model. The project team sees this approach as an effective introduction to self-assessment, which will promote a wider dialogue of organizational issues and act as a catalyst toward significant process improvement.

Building the Partnership

Initial work on the collaboration started with a series of preliminary meetings between various members of staff from NYLA and the CfBE. These meetings explored the complementary nature of the work and experiences of each team. Information sharing related to diagnostic benchmarking and experiences using the EFQM excellence framework. The clear advantages of the collaborative partnership emerged and was further developed through a NYLA/CfBE Partnership-Building Day. The NYLA team presented more detailed background of the NHS environment and their work in business excellence. The CfBE presented details of how Service PROBE (PROmoting Business Excellence) was being used in other service organizations and its links with the (EFQM) excellence framework. The day allowed for a very useful exchange of views and confirmed the potential of using the Service PROBE tool as an introduction to excellence within NHS Trusts. A number of actions were agreed upon. First, it was recognized that some changes in the "business speak" of Service PROBE was required to ensure better understanding and acceptance by NHS staff. It was also agreed that an introductory presentation was required to "sell" the idea of diagnostic benchmarking and the benefits of excellence to NHS staff. Finally, a number of NHS organizations were identified as pilot sites to test a modified version of the instrument. The aims of the project were then agreed upon and formalized.

Aims of the Collaboration

The overall aim of the collaboration is to assist NHS managers and clinicians to assess their practices and performance against the standards of "business excellence" and to plan and implement improvements. Specifically the initial project aims were:

- To develop a learning partnership between staff from NYLA and CfBE;
- To further develop the Service PROBE diagnostic benchmarking tool for use in NHS Trust organization settings;
- To work jointly in the provision and delivery of development events, known as "The Strategic Team Learning Partnership" and "The Operational Team Learning Partnership";
- To present and facilitate introductory workshops, including preparation for the deployment of PROBE for Health Care with NHS teams; and
- To facilitate the PROBE for Health Care benchmarking days for these organizations and to provide written reports of strengths and areas for improvement.

Development of the Diagnostic Tool

The Service PROBE diagnostic tool was borne out of a number of international studies including the "Made in Europe" and "Achieving World-Class Service" studies [8–12]. Service PROBE is managed in the United Kingdom by the Center for Business Instruction (CBI). The CfBE manages the PROBE scheme in the northeast of England, operating in partnership with, and on behalf of, the CBI. The Service PROBE model is based upon the premise that "Excellent Leadership creates an environment in which the organization's People contribute to their full potential, deploying effective and efficient Service Processes and Managing Performance in order to ensure the achievement of optimal Results" (Service PROBE).

The central hypothesis of Service PROBE is that better practice leads to superior performance. The same links can be found in the EFQM excellence framework, where excellence in the "enablers" leads to superior "results." The overall aims of the EFQM framework are based on the premise that "Excellent results with respect to Performance, Customers,

Figure 8.1
The Relationship between PROBE and the EFQM Excellence Model

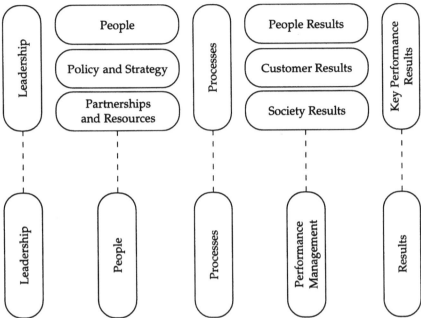

People, and Society are achieved through Leadership driving Policy and Strategy, People, Partnerships and Resources and Processes" (EFQM).

The Service PROBE tool has been designed to measure practice and performance in five broad areas: leadership, people, processes, performance management, and results. Figure 8.1 shows how this structure maps against the EFQM excellence framework.

Discussion among project team members led to revisions of Service PROBE. These revisions are primarily changes to the language used in the questions and guidance notes. The project team believes that the underlying measures remain intact, which means that the original scales and indices have been preserved. This is an important point, as it allows each new diagnostic assessment to be compared with other service organizations in the existing Service PROBE database. This comparison against an international sample of service organizations provides a rich source of "best practice," which can be drawn upon by any NHS organization in gap analysis and target setting for future improvement activities. It also provides valuable information about sectoral differences and gives strong indication of where to begin looking for exemplar organizations as potential process benchmarking partners.

The PROBE for Health Care diagnostic process is designed to help

NHS organizations gain better awareness of the principles of excellence and the context in which it can work for them. The diagnostic process allows NHS teams to share experiences in practices and performance, carefully questioning the way they deliver their services. It brings leaders and their teams together to gain better understanding of key processes. It asks them to consider how well processes work toward delivering clinically effective care and how these processes are reviewed and improved. The team gains new insight into customer-supplier interfaces, internal as well as external. They consider and question the appropriateness of the measures they use as well as the measures themselves. It requires them to carefully examine whether what they do results in satisfied patients, satisfied staff, and satisfied health commissioners.

Diagnostic Workshop Methodology

Four pilot PROBES for Health Care have been conducted with NHS organizations. In each case, the process was jointly facilitated by staff from CfBE and NYLA. During each pilot study any comments on language, understanding, or the workshop process were recorded. These comments and other qualitative data are currently being reviewed before the final version of the instrument is agreed upon.

The methodology used during a diagnostic workshop differs only slightly to that used in the original Service PROBE process. The process starts with a team of between 8 to 10 staff selected from various departments and different management and staff levels. The team is chosen to give a good spread of views across the organization. The team is briefed by the PROBE facilitator who explains the aims of the process and clarifies how they should complete the questionnaire (comprising 91 questions). The team is asked to seek out views of other colleagues within their own area of work. After the briefing, team members return to their departments and complete the questionnaire. About a week or so later, the team again meets with the PROBE facilitator. The range of scores is fully discussed and key issues of debate are recorded until the team reaches a consensus on each score. This facilitation usually lasts three to four hours and provides a unique opportunity for staff members to discuss many issues, which would not ordinarily be possible. Key issues are noted by the facilitator and are subsequently included in the final written feedback report. At the end of the day the facilitator completes an initial analysis of the results and verbally presents the key findings and benchmarking comparisons with other organizations from the PROBE database. The facilitator then follows up with a full written feedback report about a week later. The written report contains a complete assessment of the trust's "strengths" and "areas for improvement" comparing their practices and performances against the international database of service organizations. Also given are various indices comparing the trust in detail with other health and public sector organizations.

It is recommended that the trust team should meet again to discuss the findings of the written feedback report, agree upon priorities, and begin planning for action. This meeting usually takes place with a NYLA advisor and a CfBE facilitator present. Typically, this meeting will lead to further examination and improvement of those processes that have been identified as "areas for improvement." Some immediate improvements may be possible through internal improvement team activities or by the introduction of new systems. However, other improvements may need more study and analysis, and one possible way forward is to begin process benchmarking. This requires in-depth mapping and measurement of processes, and identification of other organizations (not just NHS) that are willing to share practices. Process benchmarking projects have already begun as a result of this pilot.

Case NHS Organizations

PROBE for Health Care is a strictly confidential process. The data collected during the diagnostic, the feedback report, and the benchmark comparisons are available only to the organization's PROBE team. The raw data collected from each NHS organization will be used to increase the size of the PROBE benchmarking database for future (anonymous) comparisons. The four NHS organizations participating in the pilot have agreed to be named in this chapter. Their individual results and actions are not reported here to maintain confidentiality. However, some unattributed outcomes from the work are given.

South Tees Acute Health NHS Trust (STAHT) Pathology Division

South Tees Acute Hospitals NHS Trust is based in Middlesbrough and provides health care from its three main sites for around 350,000 people living in the local authority areas of Middlesbrough, Redcar, and Cleveland. The STAHT Pathology Division provides high quality diagnostic and monitoring service to the trust, surrounding general practitioners (GPs), and other local hospitals. During 1998–1999, for the third year running, the division was rated the most cost-effective laboratory in the country. The division employs 140 staff and handles more than 1 million requests per year. To ensure good cross-hierarchical representation, their PROBE team of 12 staff was made up of managers, scientific staff, a consultant, biochemists, administration, and support staff. The division is also actively involved in the trust's Developing Excellence Project.

National Health Service Executive Human Resources Directorate

The Human Resources Directorate (HRD) is one of eight directorates within the NHS Executive HQ and is based at Leeds. HRD provides resources and expertise to develop and advance the NHS policy and reform through a number of specialist functions. These functions include a NHS Development Unit, Equal Opportunities, Employment Issues, Pay and Conditions, Workforce Planning and Education, and Medical Workforce Planning. The main aims of HRD are to ensure that the NHS has a quality work force capable of meeting the government's NHS objectives, to improve the quality of working life for all staff, and to address the NHS management capacity and capabilities so that it can deliver the reforms and changes necessary. In their work HRD staff interact with a wide range of customers, including government ministers, regional offices, medical professional bodies, education bodies, NHS chief executives and managers, and public/patients/careers. The PROBE questionnaire was completed by a team of eight employees from a range of functions and levels of seniority within HRD.

York Health Services NHS Trust

York Health Services NHS Trust is a fully integrated trust delivering acute, community, and mental health services. The trust's main facility is York District Hospital, a well-equipped modern unit of 810 beds within walking distance of the city center. It also has a number of other facilities providing another 400 beds. The trust employs approximately 5,200 staff (3,500 full-time equivalents) and during 1989–1999 treated 64,400 inpatients, 203,400 outpatients, and 71,076 accidents and emergencies. The Service PROBE questionnaire was completed by a team of 12 staff.

York Mental Health Directorate

York Mental Health Directorate (part of York Health Services NHS Trust) is managed through a mental health management team. The service has approximately 600 staff (FTE) and provides care for around 5,000 patients at any point in time, with an increasing demand each year. The main site at Bootham Park Hospital houses inpatient services for general psychiatry, an elderly assessment unit, a mother and baby unit, and a special care ward. Additionally, the site also caters to outpatient and day-clinic needs for patients from across the community. Patients are referred from a wide range of sources including GPs, community psychiatric nurses, and social services. The directorate also has community teams that cater to a wide range of needs—for example, general psychiatry and a number of specialist services, including alcohol-related problems, eating disorders, psychotherapy, forensic psychiatry, child and adolescent care, and elderly services. A major driver for the directorate is to improve its outreach community services. They make use of a number of other residential and day-clinic facilities at many different sites around the York area. These provide services for both long-term and short-term care and rehabilitation needs of patients in the community. The Service PROBE questionnaire was completed by a team of nine staff from across the directorate.

Resulting Actions

What has resulted from the diagnostic process? At this stage in the project the resulting changes to practice and performance as reported by each case organization is variable. Each has convened a follow-up meeting(s) with various team members (and other staff) to consider the issues raised during the PROBE workshop and the subsequent feedback report. In each case staff from NYLA and CfBE were invited to the meeting to discuss the report findings and to help identify future actions. This prioritization of the "areas for improvement" is a fundamental next step in the process. Following these meetings, the resulting actions for change are varied. This is partly due to the time scales involved and to a great extent is dependent on their own resource availability to make change happen. Also, it clearly must be related to other priorities, initiatives, and changes that are already under way. The next section of this chapter discusses these outcomes in more detail by an analysis of the qualitative interviews conducted with staff from each of the organizations. In the best case, it is reported that there has been significant progress made in a number of operational areas. This example demonstrates what has been achieved in one organization.

A Case Outcome

Following PROBE for Health Care in this organization, members of the team met with NYLA and CfBE and were able to agree and prioritize a number of areas for improvement. Since then, they have set up action groups and have already made a number of significant changes to their work practices. They have modified their processes for logging and reporting complaints and have set up a system to ensure regular and formal review of complaint data. To improve communications (another area for improvement), they have developed a communication strategy and introduced organization briefings. Another area of concern related to people management issues. These have now been addressed through a leadership program and improved access for all junior staff to the management process. Training and development of staff was another area for improvement. They have now completed a full review of training needs for all staff. To address customer and employee issues they have introduced two staff groups, one to focus on staff satisfaction and the other to look at customer satisfaction. They have also recognized the potential benefit of using "process benchmarking" as a route to change. Process benchmarking allows them to consider different solutions by learning from other industries. They have also begun work with an external industrial partner to improve their approaches to staff training and development, career progression, and employee support and recognition. The organization states that they have found the process so useful that they intend to undergo another PROBE in summer 2001 as part of their continuous improvement program.

POST-WORKSHOP INTERVIEWS

Part of the pilot process was to conduct qualitative semi-structured interviews with staff from each of the teams participating in the pilot workshops. Interviews were conducted with each PROBE team coordinator and two team members. Additional interviews have also been conducted with two senior managers (who were not part of the team themselves, but who commissioned the work). In each case, these managers were involved in post-PROBE follow-up meetings. Both managers also collected and analyzed written feedback from each of their PROBE team members. This feedback on the team's views of the usefulness process has also been included in the following analysis and discussion.

Analysis and Discussion of Qualitative Interviews

The following section details the aggregated responses from the interviews. Content analysis [13] has been used to identify commonly held views about the benefits and negative outcomes of the diagnostic process. Some specific examples of outcomes have also been included.

First, they were asked to give views about the overall usefulness and benefits of the process. All respondents believe that the PROBE for Health Care process had been useful (or very useful) to the organization and team members. There was a good level of agreement on the following benefits. The process provided a rapid snapshot of a range of issues across the organization. It stimulated people's thinking. The cross-section of staff involved gave a broad, relevant, and unbiased set of views. It was especially helpful to hear and discuss the views of different clinical managers. It made them think carefully and focus on the patient experience. It brought different perspectives together and broke down barriers between medical and support staff. The consensus process was very useful. In more than one case it has already prompted positive action. The team's involvement and subsequent activities have served as a catalyst for further staff involvement.

On the other hand, there were some negative aspects identified. However, all respondents did not concur with these different issues. Two respondents were concerned about the amount of time it takes each team member to complete the questionnaire, particularly when they are asked to seek views from other colleagues. Individual respondents identified other issues. One felt that there was some repetition in the questionnaire. One recognized the importance of a quick follow-up with an action day, otherwise momentum is lost. They also recognized that it was desirable to plan and make resources available to carry through any actions (change) before the diagnostic event, otherwise nothing would change. It is very important (but difficult) to free up senior managers' time and allow them to be fully involved with the process. Another concern was that the process can raise staff expectations that might not be within the control of the organization and therefore cannot be fulfilled.

They were asked about any feedback they had received from their team after the PROBE day. Overall there was good agreement that most staff found the day very positive and had enjoyed taking part. Some of the comments both positive and negative are included here.

Positive comments: one day is too short—two would be better; it stimulated me by interaction with the team (a consultant); interesting, enjoyable, and extremely useful; found the process very positive; allowed us to get away from firefighting for a while.

Negative comments: too many questions; took a long time; too business oriented; exhausting; difficult to think Trust wide; not sure that anything will change as a result.

The respondents were then asked a range of questions about different aspects of the process to determine advantages and disadvantages in more detail. There was unanimous and very positive agreement that the process provided a useful forum for open and honest discussion among staff team members. In most cases, the team benefited from the process and continued to network with one another. When asked if it had helped with communications between different staff groups, all but one agreed that it had done so, but mainly only for the team members.

All but one of the respondents agreed the process had increased awareness of internal customer-supplier relationships between different departments. In one case they believed that this was a concept already well understood in the NHS. Other comments identified that it helped the team recognize the importance of collecting "hard evidence" about how (and how well) these interfaces worked.

The written feedback report provides many output charts and commentary on the key issues for the organization. All respondents felt that it was a useful document. There were positive comments regarding clarity, structure, comprehensiveness, and that it "crystallizes key issues." In addition, a few constructive comments were made on how to improve it to make it more user friendly, particularly as many of the team members were new to the principles and language of "excellence."

When asked if the PROBE had identified any areas for improvement of which the organizations were not already aware, there was a mixed set of views. Two of the organizations believed that it did not identify any new issues but that it had objectively reinforced and confirmed many suspicions. However, one of them made the point that the degree of staff involvement in the process did prompt a positive response from the organization. In the other two cases, the respondents confirmed that PROBE had informed them of new areas for attention. In one case it had identified fundamental issues regarding their approach to performance management and a need for wider ranging qualitative assessment.

There was common agreement that PROBE provided a good introduction to the principles of the EFQM Excellence Model. For many members of the team this was their first exposure to such ideas, and it helped them gain better understanding of the underlying principles. Other comments were that it had helped team members understand the relationships between aims and strategies leading to results. Another stressed that those staff involved quickly achieved a broader understanding of the context in which they work and in all of the elements of the excellence model.

There was a mixed response when asked if they had held follow-up planning meetings that had led to actual changes or improvements. Only two of the four organizations have made significant progress to date. It should be noted, however, that they were the first two organizations to complete the pilot and have therefore had the most time to take action. Of the others, one has met to discuss the findings but has not yet agreed upon plans for change. The fourth is still at the stage of digesting the feedback report and is planning a follow-up meeting with the team and senior managers.

When asked if their organizations would use PROBE for Health Care again, there was unanimous agreement that they would. One of them has already indicated that they wish to use it again in summer 2001 and that they see this as a way of monitoring progress.

They were asked if they would like to do something differently next time. There were a number of positive changes they would make. These include: do more to engage senior managers and get real ownership from the top; start the process earlier and give more time to the team to complete the questionnaire; and give the process and outcomes higher profile. Some respondents would be happy to do it again exactly as before.

Finally, they were asked if they thought that their organizations would go on to use the EFQM Excellence Model for self-assessment. One of the organizations operates within a trust that is already using and committed to it. The other three believe that they will do so at some point in the future.

CONCLUSIONS AND FUTURE WORK

Overall, the research team believes that PROBE for Health Care has proved to be a useful process and has resulted in some positive outcomes for those NHS organizations involved. The lessons learned about the instrument and the workshop process has been invaluable, and the questionnaire and guidance notes will now be finalized for use by many other healthcare organizations in their journey to excellence.

The process provides a useful forum for open and honest discussion among staff and gives a "snapshot" of different perspectives within an organization. It can help improve communications among different staff groups, at least for the team members involved, and can increase awareness of internal customer-supplier relationships.

The process provides a good introduction to the underlying principles of excellence. It is a very useful starting point for any organization at the beginning of their quality journey. If an organization is functionally managed, if they use a "check-and-correct" attitude to quality and service standards, if they are very results focused, then the approach will help team members to understand the advantages of process thinking. However, PROBE for Health Care is not just suited to organizations that are immature in their approach to quality. This pilot study has shown that even organizations that are already committed to using the excellence model and that have already developed process thinking can benefit too.

Organizations that wish to undertake diagnostic self-assessment must consider the implications carefully. They must ensure commitment from senior management and provide resources, not only during the assessment phase but also in the prioritizing, planning, and action stages that follow. Self-assessment can raise staff expectations and can act as a catalyst for change. Senior management must be aware of this and be prepared to take action and make changes as a result of the diagnostic process. At the beginning of the process, resources need to be identified and follow-up actions need to be planned for.

Following this work, the NYLA-CfBE collaboration has already scheduled a series of benchmarking workshops throughout 2001. The workshops are offered at two levels. The first is an entry-level benchmarking day, which introduces delegates to the different types of benchmarking and gives them hands-on experience of how to get started. It also explains the strengths and limitations of the approach to continuous improvement. The second-level workshop—advanced benchmarking—builds on the first. Delegates will be asked to complete some pre-work and will work in small focused groups on a specific process of interest to them. During the day they will produce a diagnostic benchmark of this critical process for their own organization.

ACKNOWLEDGMENTS

Grateful thanks for their valuable contributions to all staff from the following organizations, who took part in this research: South Tees Acute Health NHS Trust (STAHT) Pathology Division; National Health Service Executive Human Resources Directorate (HRD); York Health Services NHS Trust; and York Mental Health Directorate.

NOTES

[1] Department of Health, *The NHS Plan: A Plan for Investment: A Plan for Reform* (London: HMSO, 2000).

[2] EFQM, *Guidelines for Self-Assessment, European Quality Foundation for Quality Management* (Brussels: EFQM, 2000).

[3] Department of Health, *A First Class Service: Quality News in the New NHS* (London: HMSO, 1998).

[4] NHS Executive, *Working Together: Securing a Quality Workforce for the NHS* (London: NHSME, 1999).

[5] Prabhu, V. B., and D. J. Yarrow, "A 'Practice-Performance' Study of North-East Manufacturing and Service Sector Industry," *Northern Economic Review*, 27, Spring/Summer 1987.

[6] Yarrow, D. J., and V. B. Prabhu, "Collaborating to Compete: Benchmarking Through Regional Partnerships," *Total Quality Management*, 10(4 & 5), 1999, s793–s802.

[7] Yarrow, D. J., V. B. Prabhu, M. Appleby, M. Allen, E. Mitchell, and E. Matykiewicz, "The Competitiveness Project: Company Benchmarking—Results and Analysis," report from the University of Northumbria at Newcastle, 1999, 37 pp.

[8] Hanson, P., C. Voss, K. Blackmon, and B. Oak, "Made in Europe, A Four Nations Best Practice Study," IBM UK Ltd/London Business School, Warwick/London, 1994.

[9] Hanson, P., C. Voss, K. Blackmon, and T. Claxton, "Made in Europe 2, An Anglo-German Design Study," IBM UK Ltd/London Business School, Warwick/London, 1996.

[10] CBI, *Fit for the Future: How Competitive Is UK Manufacturing?* (London: CBI, 1997).

[11] Voss, C., K. Blackmon, R. Chase, B. Rose, and A. V. Roth, "Achieving World-

Class Service," Severn Trent plc./UK DTI/Department of National Heritage, 1997.

[12] Voss, C., K. Blackmon, R. Cagliano, P. Hanson, and F. Wilson, "Made in Europe 3—The Small Company Study—An Anglo Italian Comparison," IBM Consulting Group, 1998.

[13] Jankowicz, A. D., *Business Research Projects* (2nd ed.) (London: Open University Press, 1996).

Chapter 9

Palliative Care: An Environment That Promotes Continuous Improvement, Learning, and Innovation

Graydon Davison and Paul Hyland

INTRODUCTION

In increasingly complex, dynamic, and financially constrained environments such as hospitals, there is a need to develop innovative solutions to problems related particularly to the cost and quality of care, and to do this on an ongoing or continuous basis. Innovative teams need "hard, focused, purposeful work" requiring "diligence, persistence, and commitment" [1, p. 72]. These are the key, almost overpowering, characteristics of teams and team members in the palliative care environment. This chapter describes the capabilities needed to manage continuous innovation, radical innovations, and continuous incremental improvements in such an environment. The continuous innovation model used in the EU-funded CIMA (Center for Improvement in Medical Assistance) project [2] is used as a starting point for this research. The capabilities required to manage a complex environment such as palliative care and other dynamic healthcare environments have been identified as: managing knowledge, in terms of its acquisition, creation, and dissemination; managing information, including collection, interpretation, and communication; interdisciplinary operations; collaborative operations; managing technologies; and managing change and its effects. Using palliative care as a case study, the research describes the capabilities identified in the literature by a number of authors [3–7] and describes how these capabilities have been observed in the palliative care environment. The palliative care environment is multidisciplinary, team based, people focused, and systemically oriented, with a singular focus: an end of life experience for an individual and the members of any supportive social system that surrounds the individual. This socially based environment is part of a larger system of health care that has a high profile in the consciousness of the general population and in the politics of the day. Palliative care teams must, therefore, accommodate and manage issues such as the economics and affordability of the provision of an end-of-life experience, the management and administration of its services within the healthcare infrastructure, and the prioritization of limited resources. In its day-to-day operation, palliative care has acquired and implemented many of the attributes of high-performing knowledge-based enterprises, such as excellence in learning and multidisciplinary, cross-functional work teams, in ways that would make it the envy of highly profitable businesses. In a unique environment, where objective quantification of measures such as customer satisfaction is often meaningless, palliative care professionals have implemented innovations in processes in a highly effective way. To date, the focus for reporting the changes and innovations in palliative care has been on quality of life and medical issues rather than learning and innovation management. Understanding of innovation within this particular environment holds useful lessons for other environments within health care, the public sector, nongovernmental organizations, and business operations in general. While many businesses have struggled to implement self-regulating teams and have invested considerable resources in attempting to gain some advantage from teamwork, it appears palliative care professionals have adopted self-regulating work teams in a highly uncertain environment as the most suitable human resource structure and practice. This chapter uses a modified CIMA model and examines the organizational capabilities needed to manage innovation within the environment. In using the CIMA model the research seeks to draw together the learning in product/process innovation and the learning in patient care innovation.

HEALTH CARE: COMPLEX, FRAGMENTED, AND CHANGING

The pressures of increased patient demand and rising costs are changing health care. The reality of these pressures is manifested in a number of ways. For example, the influence of these pressures is changing the role of supervisors and healthcare delivery systems [8], and in Australia there is formal acknowledgment of the need for structural change to healthcare systems, the introduction of systemic information management techniques, and integrated whole-of-life patient care as a response to increased demand and rising patient costs [9, 10]. Both agencies note that these issues are not limited to Australia. Whole-of-life care for patients means moving away from the paradigm of episodic intervention and care. The changes occurring to healthcare delivery systems include a move from episodic care to population-based care, redefining, for example, the hospital's role to one of providing only care that cannot be provided at lesser cost in other places [11]. The shift from episodic to population-based care means that healthcare providers must change their organizational capabilities [12]. In response to the pressures of patient demand and rising costs, new concepts for the structure, delivery, and management of health care are being reported in the literature.

Changes to privately and publicly funded healthcare systems bring with them major conceptual and operational issues and challenges to the traditional working of these systems. Healthcare managers, clinical and nonclinical, are facing a conceptual challenge in the apparent shift in healthcare theory from technical to human [13]. The structural and strategic changes this implies are mirrored in such industries as financial services, telecommunications, and transportation, giving the impression that health care is becoming a commodity [14]. The key drivers of change in health care are changes in technology, changes in the structures of political governance, and the requirement for more integrated healthcare systems [13]. New healthcare agendas will introduce new types of work and new ways of working so that current levels and types of skills and knowledge may become less relevant, as will some of the systems that support interprofessional barriers [15]. For example, the introduction of total quality management to healthcare systems changes perceptions of performance and long-standing work relationships in public hospitals when the measurement of performance includes the understanding of the system's impact on the patient, in the patient's opinion. This can challenge the established expectation of some professions to be the arbiters of meaning and challenges the role of clinicians in the hospital hierarchy [16].

A primary challenge faced in the new healthcare environment is the requirement for increased multidisciplinary operations from multiple professional streams such as clinicians, generalists, technicians, technocrats, and managers. Currently, each stream will often have its own administration, situational autonomies, certainties about status and power, and expectations of particular roles in decision-making processes. As these streams interact on a daily basis, there is a display of hierarchy based on the central role of some professions in the history of the development of health care [17]. Multiple streams lead to the fragmentation of healthcare systems, reflecting the fragmentation of disciplines and professions populating the systems. This carries its own issues, primarily the dilution of effort and suboptimal application of resources, particularly intellectual capital [13]. The issue of fragmentation influences many aspects of management in the evolving healthcare systems. However, there are two that are particularly indicated in the literature: (1) the re-

quirements for coordination of services, systemic management of resources, and ongoing interaction throughout a patient's life cycle; and
(2) the requirement to maintain a useful interface with rapidly developing technologies, particularly concerning the systemic management of
information.

PALLIATIVE CARE

The palliative care environment is actively compassionate toward people approaching an end-of-life experience, their families, and supporters.
The role of this care environment is to establish and maintain a quality
of life appropriate to each patient and the patient's requirements and to
include within it people other than the patient who are willing to be
included [5]. This environment is attended by a number of clinical and
nonclinical professions including nursing, medicine, pharmacology,
physiotherapy, occupational therapy, social work, pastoral care, grief
counseling, and administration. This is a multifactorial environment
where people are the center, not diseases, where care results from the
understanding of the causes of suffering [18], and where multiprofession
teams work collegiately so that the primary issue becomes and remains
patient comfort [19]. The quality of life of people at the end of their lives
is an issue of relief of suffering, whether the cause is physical, emotional,
spiritual, known, or unknown [20]. The patient is central in the ethics,
philosophy, and practice of palliative care. The patient's end-of-life state,
and central role in efforts to manage that state, makes the patient a par-
ticipatory member of the palliative care team who maintains a level of
autonomy and control in relation to the other team members [21].

The arrival of a patient at an end-of-life experience requiring palliative
care brings the certainty that life will end, generally within a relatively
short period of time. This single fact aside, uncertainty is the basis of the
end-of-life experience. The uncertainty is generated from at least four
sources. The first is the uncertainty of the trajectory of the disease that
is the end-of-life cause [22]. The second is a caution related to issues
regarding the death of patients in care at the end of their lives. These
issues are the conception of death, personal dignity, and the making of
informed decisions on the part of the patient and the carers [23]. The
third is the likelihood that patients will specify interventions, made on
their behalf by the professionals involved, to relieve suffering, but not
necessarily to prolong life. This can provide a level of confusion and
discomfort for the healthcare professionals involved [3, 5]. This source
of uncertainty introduces the population of the patient's social, sometimes referred to as informal, support system into the palliative equation
as both an extension of the field of responsibility for the professionals
involved and a component for consideration in the patient's suffering

and sense of loss [24, 25]. The fourth is described as the difficulty of assessing outcomes of palliative care using performance indicators such as the quality of care, quality of life, quality of death, and bereavement in a system that concerns itself with a range of care covering physical, social, and spiritual aspects. This is influenced by the fact that each patient represents a unique situation that is continually changing, requiring constant reassessment [26]. In addition to these uncertainties, each patient's end-of-life experience is occurring on two distinct levels, the conscious and the unconscious, and the depth of the experience at each level varies from patient to patient.

Palliative care is an uncertain, dynamic environment with a certain conclusion. Prior to arriving at that certain conclusion, it is the uncertainty that directs all attempts to provide care. For the professions involved, this creates a working environment that requires ongoing work-based learning, governed by an uncertain direction of care that must follow a trajectory of need, of which the patient is the major informant [27]. This learning is related to the multiprofession-based efforts to preserve or achieve a particular quality of life for the patient's end-of-life experience and includes the patient and informal carers. In the quality and operations management literature, this problem-based learning is viewed as continuous improvement. This is work-based, cross-functional learning, not discipline-specific learning. The primary and necessary characteristic of this organic learning, in terms of its need to continue to grow and change to accommodate changing patient experiences, is collaboration [28]. Despite their widespread use and popularity in many types of organizations, collaborative cross-functional teams do not automatically operate or function as well as intended. In many cases, this underperformance produces economic, service, or political consequences. In palliative care, the consequences are reductions in the effectiveness of care, resulting in deterioration in quality of life of the patient and increases in the levels of uncertainty accompanying the patient. This has major implications for the carer team's group efficacy, a group's belief in its ability to perform effectively. Team members in environments with high levels of uncertainty work independently and lower the collectivism of the team. This creates a separation between group efficacy and group effectiveness. On the other hand, when uncertainty is low, team members work interdependently and there is a positive relationship between group efficacy and group effectiveness [29]. It is to the benefit of the palliative team, including the patient, to consciously work to lower the levels of uncertainty.

Collaborative cross-functional teams are often faced with issues surrounding personal interactions and commitment [30] and, as such, palliative care teams appear to have similar problems. The relationship

Figure 9.1
The CIMA Model

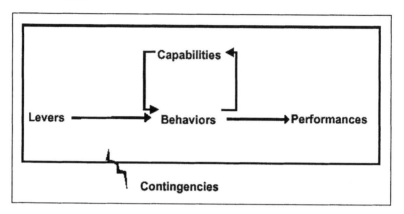

between at least two of the professions involved is perceived by many to be based on conflicting paradigms. Care and cure are paradigms basic to nursing and medicine respectively and when they conflict the result is not helpful to either outcome [31]. There is evidence that this conflict can be successfully managed but the cost is a suboptimal background to patient care, innovation, and change [32].

A CONCEPTUAL FRAMEWORK

To understand how this environment is managed and how the professions interact to achieve innovative outcomes that benefit the patient and satisfy professional paradigms, it is necessary to understand the context. This research examines the innovation process in palliative care using two starting points. The first is a definition of innovation applicable to the ethics, purpose, and focus of palliative care. This defines innovation as "the effort to create purposeful, focused change in an enterprise's economic or social potential" [1, p. 67]. The second is a conceptual framework developed as part of a study into innovation in manufacturing, the CIMA model, seen in Figure 9.1.

The CIMA model describes the relationships and learning and knowledge transfer within product innovation in terms of five interacting components that behave systemically: capabilities, levers, behaviors, performances, and contingencies [2]. The first four define a causally linked subsystem. This interacts with the fifth component, contingencies, containing variables that are generated within the subsystem and by the subsystem's environment. The interaction is also causal. This chapter describes the capabilities requisite for innovation in palliative care as described in the literature and matches these with activities observed in the palliative care environment. The remaining components will be described in future papers.

CAPABILITIES

Within the description of the components of the CIMA model, capabilities are described as integrated organizational resources, either learned through necessity or established through deliberate decisions. These resources include activities such as behaviors, skills, routines, and corporate systems and structures. Capabilities are important because they influence organizational behaviors [2]. The large cross-functional effort required to deliver palliative care mandates cross-functional and interdisciplinary capabilities. These capabilities manifest themselves in a number of ways and in the six capabilities identified so far in the literature and described in the following sections.

Managing Knowledge

Knowledge can be described as information that has been contextually processed and enriched via analysis, interpretation, and reflection [33, 34]. Knowledge has also been described as a human property, with the warning that difficulties and errors can follow an attempt to equate it with information, leading to the assumption that information technology can overcome knowledge deficiencies in organizations [35]. Knowledge contributes to organizational performance and stimulates and maintains innovative practices [33]. Managing and cultivating knowledge is a method of building, changing, displaying, and evidencing organizational competence [35]. This includes knowledge generation, capture, exploitation, and dissemination. Knowledge management in agile innovative organizations uses knowledge as the foundation of intellectual capital, in itself a major consideration in innovative environments, and should exploit an organization's internal knowledge capacity as a primary source of innovation [36], although an organization must purposefully apply its skills and knowledge to achieve successful innovation aligned to its goals [37].

Palliative care is delivered by interdisciplinary teams that include any person relevant and available to the patient's needs including family and friends of the patient [5, 24, 25]. A palliative care organization can be described as a complex, distributed organization that is fundamentally dependent on knowledge for the achievement of its primary purpose for each individual patient. The carer network that uses knowledge in this environment is widespread and multileveled. For example, the term physician can refer to a wide range of medical professionals, from family physicians to oncologists, surgeons, and pain specialists [5] for any patient, and the range will vary from patient to patient at different times in the end-of-life experience.

Each member of each patient's dynamic carer network joins the network with an existing level of knowledge and experience, an ability to learn and communicate, and has differing requirements for knowledge. An example of the range of requirements notes that cancer patients' family members caring for patients at home, and patients themselves, seek knowledge for decision making in symptom management, selection and location of treatments, use of chemotherapy, selecting a medical provider, and planning for end of life. Nurses are commonly sought as sources of this knowledge [24]. The knowledge that must be managed across and through the carer network is sometimes discipline specific, sometimes patient specific, sometimes network general, and each is always available to inform the others. This includes dissemination of knowledge throughout the carer network and the opportunistic capture and exploitation of knowledge from sources other than the carer network. The exploitation of this knowledge, to the benefit of the network, is an important part of this capability [12, 13, 27, 38].

Dynamic carer networks are rich in terms of the number and type of individuals involved. This richness is evidenced in the diversity of experience, information, intellect, biases, skills, and training that are brought to the inter- and intranetwork use and generation of knowledge [35]. There is some opinion that difficulties of measuring the effectiveness of palliative care services and treatments, with the increasing inclusion of palliative care into mainstream health care, creates a lack of knowledge that must be addressed as a matter of urgency [20]. Having the capability to manage knowledge is of primary importance to a palliative care organization.

Managing Information

Information is viewed as distinctly different from knowledge and can be described as data that have been organized and interpreted [33]. Certainly knowledge and information are linked, with information described as a knowledge precursor and foundation [39]. Knowledge is recorded, archived, and distributed and one of the primary formats or vehicles for the transport and distribution of knowledge is information [40]. However, the outcomes sought from, issues involved in, and skills necessary for managing knowledge and managing information are different. Information must be appropriately managed so that an organization can understand progress toward goals, inform the decision-making processes, and communicate to groups inside and outside of the organization [41]. In smaller, singularly focused healthcare organizations the usefulness and importance of information is related to informing the reorganization of services, policies, and structures to better suit patients and to remotely manage patients [42]. In palliative care, information has three roles, each of equal priority: it is essential to the effective operation of carers, administrators and decision makers [43]; it is a foundation of knowledge built and transferred across a number of organizational and social boundaries; and it is a vehicle for knowledge and information.

The nature of palliative care is such that a singular, coherent focus must be generated by a carer team when the object of the focus, the patient, might not be manifesting symptoms that have a singular cause. This drives a need to obtain and manage information from disparate sources within and between disciplines and dynamic carer networks and related networks in the broader healthcare community and the general community so that knowledge can be generated and utilized from situation to situation for each patient. Within the palliative care literature it is noted that effective patient care requires, among other things, useful avenues of information exchange between carers about the patient [5]. In innovation in healthcare practice, information is described as having a powerful role in evaluated intervention studies and evaluations [44]. With regard to complex organizational environments, where this is a function of the number of specialists involved and their professionalism, the diversity of backgrounds enlarges the number of information sources available for the discovery of innovations [45]. This is reflective of the rich, dynamic carer networks in palliative care. Given the multifactorial and multidisciplinary environment of palliative care and the paradigm conflicts noted in the literature, the potential for politicized information and decision-making environments exists within palliative care. Managing information is a capability fundamentally necessary to a palliative care organization.

Interdisciplinary Operations

The multifactorial nature of palliative care demands interdisciplinary operations as a capability [5, 19]. This is reflected in the general healthcare literature with discussion of the growing need for interdisciplinary education in health care as a result of the integrative approach being demanded of the new healthcare environment [12]. The usefulness of interdisciplinary operations in palliative care is the opportunity that this provides for teams to learn from one another's skills and experiences in patient care [7]. With regard to the issue of professionally based paradigm conflicts, there is a need to foster interdisciplinary discussions between medicine and nursing as a way of maintaining and strengthening communications across the paradigms [32]. This is reflected by the need within effective palliative care to remove traditional territorial thinking and interests and to raise new partnerships in the carer networks [5].

With specific regard to the management of information, multidisciplinary teams could be more effective, particularly in innovation and change if they were more effective in exchanging information within the teams [31].

Collaborative Operations

Collaboration across professional groups in health care is something beneficial that cannot be directed but can be impeded. It is capable of increasing levels of satisfaction in carers, requires common purpose, is built on trust arising from the honest communication of information, and requires the alignment of the values of the collaborators to occur successfully [6]. The operationalization of interdisciplinary collaboration in health care is dependent on the recognition of alternative perspectives on the part of the collaborators, combined with the use of communication styles that facilitate collaboration [46]. In the healthcare literature, collaboration is acknowledged as necessary and useful. The effect of low levels of collaboration on hospitals has been described in terms of organizational fragmentation with the conclusion that although hospitals may seem quite complicated, this is often a function of a lack of willingness on the part of the professions involved to collaborate [47]. The requirements of implementing vertical integration in health care mean that healthcare administrators will need to shift, conceptually and operationally, from an individual view of the world to a collaborative one [17]. The shift will mean a new vision of the delivery of healthcare services.

In palliative care, physicians, nurses, and members of other disciplines need to work collaboratively to deliver holistic care over time, to assist patients and families to come to terms with the issues of death and dying, and to move beyond the management of symptoms [7]. Community-based programs to care for the dying require the collaboration of everybody involved from the health professionals to the patients and their families [5]. Collaboration is also necessary in the creation of knowledge and the provision of information within a context such as palliative care. Knowledge is created within these communities when people with different experiences collaborate to share information collectively [48]. The relationship between collaborative operations and innovation is not well represented in the healthcare or palliative care literature.

Managing Technologies

In agile, innovative organizations technology has been characterized as knowledge applied through people, as cognitive, and as an intangible asset [36]. Technology can also be described as both the asset and the knowledge necessary to produce it [49]. Technology changes are major drivers of strategic and structural changes in health care, and technology diffusion has the ability to generate major issues such as an increased information flow and pace of activity [13]. Technologies are cited as useful in cost reduction and also as a major cause of increasing healthcare costs, with the note that technology assessment can be a highly politicized process [17, 50]. The need for management to innovate its practices so that new medical technologies can be optimally exploited therefore brings its own challenges [42]. Without technology the work of maintaining and exploiting a knowledge base of any size, as required within the new integrative healthcare environment, would be almost impossible [33]. With regard to medical innovation and its relationship to technology, the range of new medical technologies presents administrators with the dilemma of what to pay for now and what to leave until more evidence is available regarding the efficacy of the technology. This is a real issue with regard to being perceived as wasting money on less-than-useful technology or overspending on inappropriate technology. The balance between overutilization and underutilization must be appropriately struck [51].

With specific regard to palliative care, technology has been described as an enabler of the application of the ethics of care and of optimizing the utilization of comfort measures in the last days of life [3]. However, there are also concerns expressed by some healthcare professionals about the burdens provided by medical technology with relation to end-of-life patients and issues of overuse of life-sustaining technology as prolonging patient suffering [52]. The capability to manage technologies appropriately to the benefit of the palliative network is, therefore, also fundamental to successful palliative care operations.

Managing Change and the Effects of Change

A number of important changes are occurring in the general healthcare environment. One important change, not yet discussed, that has a large impact on palliative care providers is the changing status of palliative care within the healthcare environment. Concerns about increasing levels of routinization and bureaucratization that are accompanying the hospice movement's return to the mainstream healthcare environment are expressed [53]. There are particular expressions of concern that, as palliative care is returned to the healthcare mainstream, the accompanying integration of palliative physicians' expertise will remove the potential of palliation as a specialty to deliver more than symptom relief [4, 54] and that the inclusion of hospices into mainstream health care involves formalization and dehumanization of the palliative ethos, the loss of singular focus, and disillusionment among staff and volunteers of palliative organizations [21]. These are reflected in concerns that the increasing medicalization of palliative care will reduce the concept of this type of care to one of symptom management at the end of life, counter to the palliative paradigm of holistic care, bringing with it the concept that it can be measured, scrutinized, and judged in purely objective terms [18, 20]. Bringing palliative care into mainstream health care also involves reductions in nonmedical staff, and some pastoral and social workers, for example, have already lost their jobs in the name of cost efficiencies [54].

Changing demographics and increasing diversity of populations are also providing effects that must be managed. The aging of the population provides changes to the nature and needs of the dying, and there is a worldwide change of causes of death from acute conditions to chronic and progressive illnesses [7, 20]. An increasingly informed and educated patient population is demanding the consideration of alternative or complementary therapies [12]. Palliative care, while traditionally linked to cancer, has an application to other types of conditions such as AIDS, end-stage cardiovascular and pulmonary disease, and diabetes—diseases that have limited curative treatments. The inference drawn is that the scope of palliative applications is growing as the population ages [5]. The growing diversity of populations is also an issue of concern as it changes the nature and occurrence of illness and disease, which requires that the populations of the palliative care professions and the populations of the carer networks change to accommodate the new diversity [12]. The requirement of palliative carers to accommodate these changes indicates that the management of change and its effects is a critical capability. The changes occurring in palliative care have the ability to fundamentally shift its purpose. The capability to manage them should be of primary concern.

CASE STUDY

The following is a summary of observations made in 1999. The observations relate to a palliative care hospice and associated palliative care providers. In the case reported here the inclusion of a patient and an informal carer into a formal network of care within a palliative environment appears an operation of some subtlety. The first interaction with the palliative network is one of information exchange and relationship building. If, as in the case reported here, the patient is under care at home, the first encounter is with a community nurse. The role of this nurse is to manage a distributed carer network. To accomplish this, the community nurse must have the active involvement and cooperation of the patient and the patient's social support system, sometimes referred to as informal carers. Informal carers are those members of the patient's family or social network willing to provide care and comfort on a full-time basis. The initial interaction with the community nurse involves the exchange of information about assets and technologies available to the patient, assets and technologies available to the palliative care network, and the social relationship between the patient and the informal carers.

Assets and technologies available to the patient cover a wide range and can be grouped into two categories: assets and technologies available from and owned by the palliative care network and assets and technologies available from and owned by or related to the patient's personal network. Examples of the first group can be further broken down to clinical and nonclinical. Clinical assets and technologies include medications, diagnostic technologies, medical and nursing expertise and advice, accommodation at a palliative care institution, and medical and nursing care. Nonclinical assets and technologies include social workers, pastoral care workers, occupational therapists, communications, transport to and from parts of the palliative network, and advice and expertise concerning the nonclinical aspects of the end-of-life experience.

Assets and technologies available to the palliative network from the patient's side can also be broken down into two groups. The first contains the patient's views, interpretations, feelings, concerns, and opinions on a range of matters from the efficacy of medications to the ability of informal carers to personally manage the end-of-life experience. The second is the patient's own assets and technologies such as communications, layout of the home to accommodate mobility, availability of personal transport, relationship between informal carers and the patient, and the ability of informal carers to manage components of the end-of-life experience.

The community nurse must assess the balance of these groups of assets and technologies and decide whether, on balance, the best use of these is in care at home or care at an institution and, if care at home is chosen, whether the necessary relationships between these assets and technologies can be sustainably maintained. It is at this initial meeting that the patient and informal carers become part of, not subjects of, the palliative care network. Primary evidence of this is the informal carer's designated role in managing the patient's medication regime and monitoring the patient's reactions to medication. It becomes the informal carer's job to communicate variations to nominated points in the palliative network and to initially attempt to manage breakdowns in the effectiveness of medications. Characteristic of the management of this distributed network of care by the community nurse were honesty in information communicated and access to informed sources. Any question received an honest answer, regardless of whether the answer was palatable to the carer. This was particularly important in the case of the informal carer, as misinformed or uninformed persons in this position could waste the network's assets by frequent communications to check patient reactions and/or behaviors. Questions asked and answered included expectations for the end-of-life experience, time frames, symptoms, and behavioral changes to be expected on the part of the patient and the informal carer. All of the palliative network's information sources, clinical and nonclinical, are made available to the patient and the informal carer. Sources of information on clinical aspects of care were available twenty-four hours per day. It is worth noting that a community nurse manages a number of these distributed networks simultaneously and that the assessments of the viability of each network occur at each visit. Viability assessments are also made at each contact with the palliative network. In both cases, the patient and the informal carer are used as informed sources of information.

Upon admission to a palliative care institution, the care delivery process moves from a widely distributed network to a more narrowly distributed network. The assets and technologies owned by the palliative institution begin to predominate where, before, the patient's assets and technologies had been predominant. It is at this point that the distributed palliative network, which has been behaving primarily as an information transfer system via the community nurse, appears more as a pool of disciplines and experience from which the palliative care team that accompanies the patient to the end of life forms to meet the patient's needs. The frequency of interaction with members of the palliative network rises dramatically, but not to the detriment of the role of the patient or the informal carer. An important note here is that the size of the role of the patient and informal carer is to some extent voluntary and, up to the point at which it becomes a clinical hindrance, the palliative network will attempt to accommodate the role choices made and the resulting behaviors. Expectations become a primary asset on the patient's side. Nonclinical and clinical members of the palliative network seek expectations of the palliative experience from the patient and informal carer. Nonclinical components such as spirituality, beliefs, faith, relationships, feelings, and concerns become more openly discussed as the palliative network attempts to understand the patient's approach to, views on, and requirements of these things. Within this narrowly distributed network of care, where palliative assets and technologies are closer to hand and the end-of-life experience is nearer and more real, the palliative network strives for balance in the clinical and nonclinical aspects of the patient's life, letting the patient set the balance.

During this time, the primary interactions among the patient, informal carer, and the palliative network are through nurses. As well as care, nurses provide information on topics ranging from the availability of spare pillows to the timing of the registrar's rounds, expected reactions to changes in medications and, on occasion when pressed privately by the informal carer, behaviors that could be expected at the end of life.

This last information was always given after the point had been made that the end of life was an individual experience for each patient and could vary greatly among patients. The point was also made that the same applies to informal carers, family members, and other members of the patient's social network. All communications with members of the palliative network are frank and informative, so that no information is withheld. The same rule applies as it did in the distributed network: lack of information or the provision of misinformation waste network resources as people attempt to track information along the wrong paths.

Within the narrowly distributed network of the palliative institution, as the end of life draws closer and the patient's demands on the institution's assets and technologies grow more frequent, it is more common to see a small multidisciplinary team of carers than an individual carer. The most common team of this type is registrar and nurse, sometimes registrar, nurse, and nurse unit manager. It is not uncommon also to see registrar, nurse, and pain specialist. Nurses more frequently attend in pairs because of the patient's mobility problems. During this time the informal carers are an active part of the carer team. The relationship with the patient is used to help interpret for and discuss with the patient, patient management issues ranging from changes to the symptom management regime to the need for the patient to maintain dietary intake. The informal carer is used to help explain the patient's circumstances to the patient and to explain the patient's concerns and reactions to the formal carers.

When a mixed carer team comes together with the patient, the normal clinical hierarchy, doctor in charge, is reflected. During these discussions between patient, informal carer, and the mixed carer teams it is not uncommon to observe the team leadership change as the understanding of the patient's condition, physical symptoms, or family concerns change. This is often manifested by the discipline no longer necessary to the situation, for example the registrar, leaving the situation after a formal acknowledgment that the discipline could not contribute to a resolution at the time and that another team member was in charge of the particular situation. The leadership of the team is governed by the patient's need.

DISCUSSION AND CONCLUSION

The capabilities described in the literature are reflected in the case study to varying degrees. The original interaction between the patient and the palliative network, via the community nurse, was an information-gathering and knowledge-generating exercise for each individual involved. The distinction between knowledge and information is observable. Information is swapped between the carer network and the patient's network regarding, for example, availability of resources such as advice, support, and medication. Using this information, knowledge is generated on the part of the patient and informal carer about the capability of the carer network to remotely support the patient and informal carer in the home-based situation. On the part of the community nurse, knowledge is created and recorded about the capability of the patient's resources to support the home-based situation and to utilize the remote support mechanisms of the palliative network. The community nurse applies the information provided to the context for discussion and to personal experience to produce an assessment of capabilities related to the context. Knowledge is generated.

The frequency of observable applications of interdisciplinary operations and collaborative operations increases as the timing of the patient's end of life becomes more apparent. The closing of the end of life brings an increase in some of the accompanying uncertainties such as expected behaviors at the end of life, expectations of symptoms, expectations of time frames, and the behaviors of actual symptoms. The attempt to address these uncertainties becomes more observably interdisciplinary and collaborative because multiple uncertainties begin to present themselves in conjunction and they appear to become more interactive. This requires their management to be interdependently organized. On being presented with a multicausal effect, the end of life, the carer network provides a multiskilled response. While this is the case throughout the patient's interaction with the palliative system, it becomes more frequent as the patient's uncertainties begin to occur in parallel. It also becomes apparent that neither interdisciplinary nor collaborative operations always require the physical presence of a representative of each discipline.

The capability of accommodating and managing technologies is present. A broad range of technologies is utilized. The community nurse is required to assess and balance the efficacy of the technologies available on the patient's part and those available on the palliative network's part while the patient remains at home. Patient's notes are recorded by members of individual disciplines. These same disciplines are also involved in the assessment of other technologies as aids to symptom diagnosis and management. The pain specialist used a simple pain scale (asked of the patient) with the observations and experiences of the attending nurses plus the specialist's own observations and experiences, plus the patient's records to modify or maintain a pain management regime. If necessary, the pharmacologist will adjust dosages, issue new drugs, and record the changes. In an effort to understand causes of changing or new symptoms, the patient will be sent to a nearby hospital for appropriate diagnostic tests, for example X-rays, Magnetic Resonance Imaging, Computer Aided Tomography, or ultrasound. The technology employed depends on the suspected causes.

The capability of managing change and the effects of change was not

Figure 9.2
The CIMA Model in Palliative Care

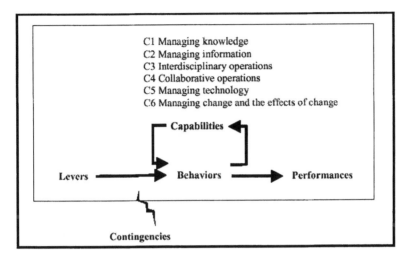

observed, although anecdotal evidence exists that there are concerns among the staff about the effects on palliative care of its absorption into the general healthcare system.

Since capabilities are the focus of this chapter, many of the descriptions of capabilities found in the literature are accompanied by descriptions of behaviors necessary to support the capabilities, and this is reflected within this chapter. In addition, behaviors supporting capabilities were observed and identified in the case study. The link is described in the literature, as it is in the CIMA model. Currently it is proposed that the CIMA model of innovation management in palliative care can be depicted by Figure 9.2.

Capabilities appearing in the original CIMA model were: knowledge generation; learning alignment; knowledge transfer and diffusion; and knowledge retailing [2]. While the capabilities in product innovation and palliative care are not identical, there are substantial similarities.

Palliative care is an innovative environment containing useful lessons that can be understood and communicated to a wider audience. These lessons can be investigated, understood, and communicated in the language of management, using analytical tools such as the CIMA methodology. This chapter has described some capabilities necessary for the management of innovation in palliative care networks from the general healthcare, palliative care, and management literature as well as from observations of a palliative network in operation. The chapter has examined the usefulness of an investigative framework for relating capabilities, learning behaviors, organizational levers, and performances within a contingency-driven environment. Initial results indicate that the framework is useful in the palliative care environment. Further investigations are planned. These will provide a richer description of the management and exploitation of innovation in palliative care, using the CIMA model as the framework for the description of the interrelationships among the necessary capabilities, learning, and other behaviors that support the capabilities, the levers that are used to guide and influence innovation management, and the performances that results from the application of the these components. This will be described within and related to a contingency-driven environment.

NOTES

[1] Drucker, P. F., "The Discipline of Innovation," *Harvard Business Review*, May–June 1985, 67–72.

[2] Gieskes, J.F.B., and I.W.H.A. Langenberg, "Learning and Improvement in Product Innovation Processes: Enabling Behaviors," Proceedings INCOSE Conference (International Council on Systems Engineering), Minneapolis, MN, July 16–20, 2000.

[3] Henkelman, W. J., and P. M. Dalinis, "A Protocol for Palliative Care Measures," *Nursing Management*, 29(1), 1998, 40–46.

[4] Kearney, M., "Palliative Medicine—Just Another Speciality?" *Palliative Medicine*, 6, 1992, 39–46.

[5] McDonald, J., and J. Krauser, "Toward the Provision of Effective Palliative Care in Ontario," in Latimer, E. (Ed.), Excerpts from OMA Colloquium on Care of the Dying Patient, 1996.

[6] Liedtka, J. M., E. Whitten, and J. S. Jones, "Enhancing Care Delivery Through Cross-Disciplinary Collaboration: A Case Study," *Journal of Healthcare Management*, 43(2), 1998, 185–205.

[7] Witt Sherman, D., "Training Advanced Practice Palliative Care Nurses," *Generations*, 23(1), 1999, 87–90.

[8] McConnell, C. R., The "Evolving Role of the Healthcare Supervisor: Shifting Paradigms, Changing Perceptions, and Other Traps," *Health Care Supervisor*, 15(1), 1996, 1–11.

[9] New South Wales Health Department, *A Framework for Managing the Quality of Health Services in New South Wales*, State Health Publication No. (HPA) 990024, 1999.

[10] New South Wales Health Council, Report of the NSW Health Council, "A Better Health System for New South Wales," 03/2000, New South Wales Department of Health, 2000.

[11] Henderson, M. D., "Operations Management in Health Care," *Journal of Health Care Finance*, 21(3), 1995, 44–47.

[12] Heller, B. R., M. T. Oros, and J. Durney-Crowley, "The Future of Nursing Education: 10 Trends to Watch," *Nursing and Health Care Perspectives*, 21(1), 2000, 9–13.

[13] Grantham, C. E., L. D. Nichols, and M. Schonberner, "A Framework for the

Management of Intellectual Capital in the Healthcare Industry," *Journal of Health Care Finance*, 23(3), 1997, 1–19.

[14] Keaney, M., "Are Patients Really Consumers?" *International Journal of Social Economics*, 26(5), 1999, 149–160.

[15] Connelly, J., T. Knight, C. Cunningham, M. Duggan, and J. McClenahan, "Rethinking Public Health: New Training for New Times," *Journal of Management in Medicine*, 13(4), 1999, 210–217.

[16] Hansson, J., "Quality in Health Care: Medical or Managerial?" *Managing Service Quality*, 10(2), 2000, 357–361.

[17] Newhouse, Robin P., and M. E. Mills, "Vertical Systems Integration," *Journal of Advanced Nursing*, 29(10), 1999, 22–29.

[18] Barbato, M., "Palliative Care in the 21st Century—Sink or Swim," *Newsletter of the New South Wales Society of Palliative Medicine*, May 1999

[19] Meyers, J. C., "The Pharmacist's Role in Palliative Care and Chronic Pain Management," *Drug Topics*, 141(1), 1997, 98–107.

[20] Higginson, I. J., "Evidence Based Palliative Care," *British Medical Journal*, 319(7208), 1999, 462–463.

[21] McGrath, P., "A Spiritual Response to the Challenge of Routinization: A Dialogue of Discourses in a Buddhist-Initiated Hospice," *Qualitative Health Research*, 8(6), 1998, 801–812.

[22] Rose, K., "A Qualitative Analysis of the Information Needs of Informal Carers of Terminally Ill Cancer Patients," *Journal of Clinical Nursing*, 8(1), 1999, 81–88.

[23] Pierce, S., "Allowing and Assisting Patients to Die: The Perspectives of Oncology Practitioners," *Journal of Advanced Nursing*, 30(3), 1999, 616–622.

[24] Lewis, M., V. Pearson, S. Corcoran-Perry, and S. Narayan, "Decision Making by Elderly Patients with Cancer and Their Caregivers," *Cancer Nursing*, 20(6), 1997, 389–397.

[25] Rose, K, "How Informal Carers Cope with Terminal Cancer," *Nursing Standard*, 11(30), 1997, 39–42.

[26] Rose, K, "Palliative Care: The Nurse's Role," *Nursing Standard*, 10(11), 1995, 38–44.

[27] Henkelman, W. J., and P. M. Dalinis, "A Protocol for Palliative Care Measures—Part 2," *Nursing Management*, 29(2), 1998, 36C–36G.

[28] Jassawalla, A. R., and H. C. Sashittal, "Building Collaborative Cross-Functional New Product Teams," *Academy of Management Executive*, 13(3), 1999, 50–63.

[29] Gibson, C. B., "Do They Do What They Believe They Can? Group Efficacy and Group Effectiveness Across Tasks and Cultures," *Academy of Management Journal*, 42(2), 1999, 138–152.

[30] Mintzberg, H., J. Jorgensen, D. Dougherty, and F. Westley, "Some Surprising Things about Collaboration—Knowing How People Connect Makes It Work Better," *Organizational Dynamics*, 25(1), 1996, 60–71.

[31] Oughtibridge, D., "Under the Thumb," *Nursing Management*, 4(8), 1998, 22–24.

[32] Krishnasamy, M., "Nursing, Morality, and Emotions: Phase I and Phase II Clinical Trials and Patients with Cancer," *Cancer Nursing*, 22(4), 1999, 251–259.

[33] Duffy, J., "Knowledge Management: What Every Information Professional Should Know," *Information Management Journal*, 34(3), 2000, 10–16.

[34] Davenport, T. H, D. E. De Long, and M. C. Beers, "Successful Knowledge Management Projects," *Sloan Management Review*, 39(2), 1998, 43–57.

[35] Brown, J. S., and P. Duguid, "Organizing Knowledge," *California Management Review*, 40(3), 1998, 90–111.

[36] Pérez-Bustamante, G., "Knowledge Management in Agile Innovative Organizations," *Journal of Knowledge Management*, 3(1), 1999, 6–17.

[37] Pitt, M., and K. Clarke, "Competing on Competence: A Knowledge Perspective on the Management of Strategic Innovation," *Technology Analysis and Strategic Management*, 11(3), 1999, 301–316.

[38] Cowling, A., K. Newman, and S. Leigh, "Developing a Competency Framework to Support Training in Evidence-Based Health Care," *International Journal of Health Care Quality Assurance*, 12(4), 1999, 149–160.

[39] Abell, A., "Skills for Knowledge Environments," *Information Management Journal*, 34(3), 2000, 33–41.

[40] Berman Brown, R., and M. J. Woodland, "Managing Knowledge Wisely: A Case Study in Organizational Behavior," *Journal of Applied Management Studies*, 8(2), 1999, 175–198.

[41] Myburgh, S., "The Convergence of Information Technology and Information Management," *Information Management Journal*, 34(2), 2000, 4–16.

[42] Alemi, F., "Management Matters: Technology Succeeds When Management Innovates," *Frontiers of Health Services Management*, 17(1), 2000, 17–30.

[43] Austin, J. C., K. D. Hornberger, J. E. Shmerling, and M. W. Elliot, "Managing Information Resources: A Study of Ten Healthcare Organizations," *Journal of Healthcare Management*, 45(4), 2000, 229–239.

[44] Tolson, D., "Practice Innovation: A Methodological Maze," *Journal of Advanced Nursing*, 30(2), 1999, 381–390.

[45] Frambach, R. T., "An Integrated Model of Organizational Adoption and Diffusion of Innovations," *European Journal of Marketing*, 27(5), 1993, 22–41.

[46] Van Ess Coeling, H., and P. L. Cukr, "Communication Styles that Promote Perceptions of Collaboration, Quality, and Nurse Satisfaction," *Journal of Nursing Care Quality*, 14(2), 2000, 63–74.

[47] Mintzberg, H., "Toward Healthier Hospitals," *Health Care Management Review*, 22(4), 1997, 9–18.

[48] Amidon, D. M., "Blueprint for 21st Century Innovation Management," *Journal of Knowledge Management*, 2(1), 1998, 23–31.

[49] Archibugi, D., and R. Simonetti, "Objects and Subjects in Technological Interdependence. Towards a Framework to Monitor Innovation," *International Journal of the Economics of Business*, 5(3), 1998, 295–309.

[50] Friedman, L. H., J. B. Goes, and R. Orr, "The Timing of Medical Technology Acquisition: Strategic Decision Making in Turbulent Environments," *Journal of Healthcare Management*, 45(5), 2000, 317–331.

[51] Moskowitz, D. B., "The Trouble with Medical Innovation," *Business and Health*, 17(5), 1999, 38–42.

[52] Schwarz, J. K., "Assisted Dying and Nursing Practice," *Journal of Nursing Scholarship*, 31(4), 1999, 367–373.

[53] Rasmussen, B. H., and P. O. Sandman, "How Patients Spend Their Time in a Hospice and in an Oncological Unit," *Journal of Advanced Nursing*, 28(4), 1998, 818–828.

[54] Kelleher, M., "Health Promoting Palliative Care: What's 'Psychosocial' Got to Do with It?" *Newsletter of the New South Wales Society of Palliative Medicine*, May 1999.

Chapter 10

Quality of Care: Reductions in Health Care for Clinically Ineffective Services

Carol Davies and Paul Walley

INTRODUCTION

Little is known about how decisions are made to either reduce or stop health services that are known to be clinically ineffective. There is a well-recognized delay in the publication of research findings and uptake into practice [1–4]. Some procedures may become part of established practice although no formal evaluation of effectiveness has been carried out [5]. There is an assumption that release of resources from clinically ineffective services will be available for services that are known to be effective, thus improving quality for patients.

There have been moves over the last decade to establish formal, systematic ways of informing clinicians and health service managers about clinical effectiveness and cost effectiveness evidence so that professionals and managers can ensure practice reflects the best available research. Many initiatives, such as the international Cochrane Collaboration, critically evaluate evidence and their findings are made available using new IT technologies. These are more easily accessible by clinicians and managers than paper-based dissemination methods, with the proviso that users have access to new technologies. However, even when good evidence is easily available, individuals and organizations may be slow to act upon research findings, and reduction initiatives may not always be successful.

This study was undertaken to gather evidence of changes that have been successfully or unsuccessfully implemented in the United Kingdom and internationally over the last 10 years and to identify critical factors relating to either success of failure of reduction attempts.

METHOD

Opinion Sampling

Identification of reduced health services and factors affecting reduction decisions in the United Kingdom and internationally over the last 10 years, for both successful and unsuccessful change, were initially identified by opinion sampling. In the United Kingdom, opinion sampling in the West Midlands (population 5,335,600) included initial telephone interviews with key decision makers, such as directors and chief executives of healthcare providers and healthcare purchasers in the National Health Service (NHS). Types of NHS organizations included health authorities, acute hospital trusts, community trusts, and primary care trusts. International opinion sampling sought views via e-mail discussion groups; questionnaires distributed at the 16th Annual Meeting of the International Society of Technology Assessment in Health Care (ISTAHC), The Hague, Netherlands, 2000; and via personal contacts around the world.

Qualitative Case Studies

In the West Midlands, once NHS organizations had been identified as attempting some kind of reduction, successful and unsuccessful organizations from the same type of organization and attempting the same reduction were compared through detailed, qualitative case studies. These involved face-to-face interviews with other representatives of the organization, usually people closely involved with managing or delivering the particular service identified. Internationally, in-depth face-to-face or telephone interviews were conducted with key representatives of government officials or health service representatives.

Literature Review

Published evidence of international reduction attempts was identified through a literature review.

Data Analysis

Qualitative data analysis identified common themes in successful and unsuccessful reduction attempts both in the United Kingdom and internationally.

RESULTS

West Midlands, United Kingdom Survey Responses

Information was obtained from 38 organizations from a total of 60 health authorities, acute and community trusts (63% response rate) plus 15 primary care trusts from a total of 61 (25% response rate) in the West Midlands.

International Survey Responses

Detailed information from Brazil, Egypt, India, Malaysia, France, the United States and Canada was obtained from government representatives of health services and practitioners.

Service Reductions (United Kingdom)

Clinical services identified as successfully or unsuccessfully reduced in the United Kingdom are shown in Table 10.1. Two of the four unsuccessful reduction attempts had been achieved in some organizations but not others. In particular, the unsuccessful prescribing attempt had relied on pharmaceutical company employees to implement change. Most attempted reductions were successful.

As part of national major service reorganizations, there has been a shift from acute to primary or community care in certain sectors. These major changes were undertaken as a result of national policy decisions relating to perceived effectiveness of service delivery rather than decisions by individual trusts based on research evidence of effectiveness for specific clinical conditions. For example, after the 1990 Community Care Act, there was a move from acute to community or primary care in mental health services and in 2000 to 2001, following the abolition of fund-holding, the reorganization of primary care administration and management into trusts. Such changes have had wide-reaching effects and illustrate the need to distinguish between effectiveness of a specific treatment (i.e., proven effectiveness to relieve or cure a clinical condition) and, alternatively, the (cost) effectiveness of service delivery to identifiable groups of patients.

Respondents were aware of literature evidence for treating individual clinical conditions, but often there were other factors influencing change, such as the need for efficiency savings: "We don't have the [nursing] resources to keep doing everything, so it becomes even more imperative that what people do is sound." All services identified were partial reductions and a few respondents made it clear that although method of

Table 10.1
West Midlands, United Kingdom: Successful and Unsuccessful Service Reductions

Clinical Service/Treatment	Outcomes in Different Organizations
grommets	successful
wisdom teeth extraction	successful
varicose vein surgery	successful
tonsillectomy	successful
sterilization reversal	successful
change in leg ulcer treatment	successful
barium meals	successful
thrombolytic therapy in coronary heart disease (*increased for infarction*)	successful
family planning/sterilization and reversal	successful
palliative care	successful
hearing tests in children (*universal distraction test to electronic test, targeted groups only*)	successful
family planning clinics	successful
prescribing in primary care	successful/unsuccessful
D&C in women < 40 years	successful/partially successful/unsuccessful
inguinal hernia (*open to laprascopic*)	unsuccessful
in-vitro fertilization treatment	unsuccessful

delivery had been changed, sometimes due to improved technology, there had been no real cuts in services. There was a clear difficulty in matching the existing evidence to the changes at the local level, often because evidence was unclear or in some instances contradictory. In addition, change was perceived as difficult due to resistance from individuals or groups and patient expectations. "On the one hand, we have evidence from analytic research, of which by definition the greatest internal validity is achieved by randomized controlled trial, and on the other, we have patients and clinicians whose problems and interactions are complex and cannot be reduced to 'pure' questions which can be unequivocally answered by 'pure' high quality, high in the hierarchy, evidence." There was also a clear preference for nationally directed guidelines on what should be changed, but it was noted that directions on how to achieve change were never identified: "Where National Service Frameworks are in place then that is obviously the basis on which one moves."

While changes in service delivery had the most far-reaching effects, no one could quantify whether or not this had saved any money. It was also unlikely that evidence was systematically collected to identify any kind of saving from reductions. Decision making was always carried out by groups, sometimes with patient representatives, and in the words of one interviewee, "It is not possible within the health service for an individual to take the decision [to reduce a service]." Decisions were not necessarily easy and were rarely quick. The average time to implement decisions fell between 6 and 24 months, but perceived speed of reduction also depended on the respondent's point of view. Change was also used as a bargaining tool by administrators and clinicians, and there was a certain weariness in attitude expressed by many respondents at the difficulties encountered on both sides.

There were transitional costs associated with all the changes identified such as retraining, new building, public information, and some redundancy payments or early retirements. No financial savings were identified. Any financial saving that had occurred was reinvested elsewhere or used to repay debt.

In implementing change it was unlikely that operational issues had been defined and there was a lack of business and management planning techniques such as business process reengineering. Exceptionally, where change methods had been more systematic, there had been a divergence of intention and results in practice.

Critical Factors in Successful Reductions (United Kingdom)

In the United Kingdom, critical success factors in reducing services included:

- Clear research evidence
- Government directives
- Efficiency savings
- Culture of change
- Wide consultation and agreement
- Training and education
- Extra funding to support the change process
- Monitoring and feedback of change

Critical Factors in Unsuccessful Reduction Attempts (United Kingdom)

Apart from a lack of critical success factors listed above, other factors included:

* Lack of experience in reduction
* Opposition by particular groups or individuals
* Patient factors such as high social deprivation
* Lack of operational issues and procedures in management of change (e.g., budgeting)
* Lack of planning for change (e.g., business process reengineering)
* Intention and practice divergence

Service Reductions (International)

Internationally, there was a clear distinction between developed and less developed countries. In the developed countries of Europe, North America, and Australia, similar services and issues were identified, comparable to those identified in the United Kingdom. Reductions in health services were usually part of health budget constraints and cutbacks. Clinicians and health administrators jointly took decisions on any reductions. In France, for example, there was major concern over funding: "The never ending and constantly increasing health insurance deficit is having economic consequences for all the people involved within the health system. Those reductions could have been avoided if the economic health of the country had been better off and unemployment reduced." French health authorities had also considered various other options, such as patients paying for some types of drugs, bandages, and tests. On a national level, reduction in quotas per physician had also been advocated in relation to prescription expenses and the total number of tests conducted per year.

In less developed countries, officially there is no reduction of health services that is undertaken on a voluntary basis or as part of the health organization's strategy. However, services are affected due to a host of other factors, (e.g., nonavailability of clinicians, nonfunctional equipment, absence of funds). This is because of the immense "social responsibility" on governments to maintain services at whatever cost. Perhaps the only region in the developing world where such reduction takes place is in Latin America. Service reductions identified from the opinion survey are shown in Table 10.2.

Some countries, such as Egypt, do not have a modern healthcare system and there is little infrastructure (medical education and monetary

Table 10.2
International Service Reductions

Country	Services Identified	Type of Change	Reason
Brazil	no official reductions but:		
	pediatrics	discontinued	shortfalls in funding
	specialized surgery (e.g., gall bladder, neurosurgery)	discontinued	shortfalls in funding
Egypt	palliative care	reduced	shortfalls in funding
	open heart surgery	reduced	shortfalls in funding
	orthopedics	reduced	shortfalls in funding
India	no official reductions but:		
	anesthetics	reduced	shortfalls in funding
	obstetrics and gynecology	reduced	shortfalls in funding
Malaysia	A&E (tertiary)	reduced	shortfalls in funding
	outpatient services (primary and secondary)	reduced	shortfalls in funding
	dentistry	reduced	shortfalls in funding
France	breast and colon cancer	reduced variations in follow-up using clinical practice guidelines	improved quality of service and inappropriate appointments
	diagnostic tests	reduced	
	prescribing	reduced	
	number of doctors	reduced	
	healthcare taxation	approximately 50% of population does not pay healthcare tax	disquiet over disproportionate payment system
	vascular tests	reduced	financial
	chemical treatment of varicose veins	reduced	financial
	surgical and nonsurgical procedures (unspecified)	reduced	financial
United States	dentistry immunization child care	reduced 35–40% overall	lower budget
Canada	blood gas measurements	reduced per patient (45% overall)	annual savings of $45,000 direct costs at one hospital

resources), although these problems are currently being addressed. The provision of health services often includes mixed public and private funding but, for example, in Malaysia, public services may be inconvenient and time consuming to use, whereas private systems are too expensive for many people. Additional types of services often exist alongside Western style medicine (e.g., Chinese, Ayurvedic, and Malay), but practitioners are not necessarily formally registered and many work part-time.

Some countries may not collect healthcare data, or data that is collected may be only from the public not private system. This results in unreliable international data, and official surveys of health care may not be undertaken. In India, for example, no official survey has been undertaken to identify the services most affected by reduction, as this can be very controversial with legal ramifications.

In the event of difficulties with services, government response strategies vary. Reduction or disruption in health services are unavoidable and may keep happening on a regular basis. In India the government does not have any specific action plan in place to avoid such recurrences, except that disciplinary action may be taken against "erring clinicians," although funds are disbursed quickly to rectify faulty equipment, for example.

Critical Factors in Reduction Attempts (International)

Critical factors in Europe, North America, and Australia were similar to those identified in the United Kingdom for successful and unsuccessful attempts, particularly factors related to finance.

Although the main critical factor in less developed countries was identified as "shortfall" in funding, it was clear that this was a very sensitive issue. Respondents were equally aware of research evidence for reduction, but it seemed as though the scale of the difficulties in providing good quality services was too great for evidence-based reductions to be clearly and openly addressed. In most cases, data or information on health states of the population may be subjective and not based on empirical evidence or research findings. The question "How are reduction decisions taken?" has little meaning in the context of less developed countries. Lack of provision and any reductions that do take place are almost always due to financial constraints. Services are also often constrained through geographical difficulties of delivering care over wide areas and to sparse populations.

DISCUSSION

There is currently great emphasis in the United Kingdom on quality assurance, part of which is clinicians' awareness and use of "best" evidence in practice [6]. However, significant findings from systematic overviews and randomized controlled trials—for example, thrombolytic therapy—do not necessarily translate automatically into practice. In research involving interventions that attempt to change practice, there is often no obvious or measurable unit of outcome. Decision making is often undertaken in a situation of uncertainty about the effectiveness and costs of interventions [7]. Our UK study highlighted the fact that research evidence is often applicable only to certain patient groups, may be conflicting and sometimes controversial, and may not be generally applicable to local situations. Although the majority of our UK respondents did not identify financial savings as the main reason for reduction, the clear preference was for any savings that do accrue from reduction to stay within the same service. There is also a productivity paradox in that consumers of health care may gain and unit costs fall, but total consumption rises, therefore no savings are made. As we found, there is normally no identifiable cost saving associated with reduction or release of resources, although redeployment or repayment of debt takes place.

The World Health Organization (WHO) describes healthcare decisions as being left to an individual country's health system to plan and manage in the manner deemed to be the best and most appropriate way. One of the key policies of WHO is "ensuring equitable access to Health Services for all." This, according to the organization, is the closest that WHO can get to ensuring that health services are not reduced and are available for one and all. However, WHO does not have any statutory or veto powers to ensure that their member countries do not reduce or rationalize health services.

CONCLUSION

Information on effective and cost-effective health care is widely available with new technologies, although access may be very limited in the less developed world. However, implementation of findings is a slow and complex process, and there remain many barriers to effective implementation of service reduction attempts in the developed world. Although finance was not identified as a key factor in the United Kingdom, it did play some part in service reductions to improve quality through reducing clinically ineffective services. In the less developed world, finance was the key factor in lack of development or provision of services. The scale of the difficulties in providing adequate services in many countries left little room for addressing reduction of particular services based on research evidence.

NOTES

[1] Dodie, J., "The Research-Practice Gap and the Role of Decision Analysis in Closing It," *Health Care Analysis*, 4, 1996, 5–18.

[2] Lomas, J., "Diffusion, Dissemination, and Implementation: Who Should Do What?" *Annals of the New York Academy of Science*, 703, 1993, 226–235.

[3] Crossthwaite, C., and L. Curtice, "Disseminating Research Results—The Challenge of Bridging the Gap Between Health Research and Health Action," in *Health Promotion International* (Oxford: Oxford University Press, 1994).

[4] Freemantle, N., and I. Watt, "Dissemination: Implementing the Findings of Research," *Health Libraries Review*, 11, 1994, 133–137.

[5] Haines, A., and A. Donald (Eds.), *Getting Research Findings into Practice* (London: BMJ Publications, 1998).

[6] Freemantle, N., J. Wood, and J. Mason, "Evaluating Change in Professional Behavior: Issues in Design and Analysis," Center for Health Economics Discussion Paper 171, University of York, 1999.

[7] Fenwick, E., K. Claxton, M. Sculpher, and A. Briggs, "Improving Efficiency and Relevance of Health Technology Assessment: The Role of Iterative Decision Analytic Modeling," Center for Health Economics Discussion Paper 179, University of York, 2000.

Part III

Emerging Technologies: Adoption, Adaptation, and Implementation

Chapter 11

Emerging Technologies: Diffusion and Quality Management of Teleconsultation Modalities in Rehabilitation

Wim H. Van Harten, Hans K. C. Bloo,
and Rob F. M. Kleissen

INTRODUCTION

Various aspects of quality management have been introduced into healthcare organizations during the last decade. The features that seem to be most widely implemented are various forms of accreditation/certification, guidelines development, and the introduction of the quality improvement circle. As quality management has both a static and dynamic side, it is interesting to observe that in practice the introduction of the static aspects—for instance, the adherence to written procedures and the implementation of guidelines—is most frequently observed. The dynamic side, which is more of a conceptual nature (continuous improvement, total quality management), seems to be more difficult to actually implement in practice.

Nevertheless, there is a relationship between the dynamic form of quality management and the realization of various innovations in healthcare technology. An adequate patient orientation leads to up-to-date information on trends and developments of the needs and demands of certain patient categories. Combined with an internal quality management system that is geared toward continuous improvement, minor and major improvements and innovations are necessarily the result.

Following this process, the actual implementation in practice will usually not be a major obstacle. New technologies that are presented to healthcare workers and institutions from outside, such as the research and development department or the international health technology forum, are faced with a different dilemma. The diffusion process of new technologies on the macro and meso levels is not just following a technical concept but is to a major extent influenced by sociodynamic reality. It is relevant to link this to the perspective of dynamic quality management in order to obtain the most effective level of implementation. In this chapter a conceptual framework is presented that can be used to observe and explain the various aspects involved in the introduction of new technologies from the perspective of quality management.

A Framework for Introduction of New Technologies Fusing the Quality Perspective

Rogers [1] has presented his theory on the diffusion of new technologies, and on the macro level it seems to be valid for health care. On the organizational level he discerns the stages of initiation (agenda setting and matching) and implementation (redefining/restructuring, clarifying and routinizing). Nevertheless, his schedule has more of a technical nature, whereas health care is provided in a service environment where most activities are performed by employees, so the human factor cannot be underestimated. And this point is not emphasized in his theory (especially for innovations *within* organizations). Therefore, his more technical and time-related schedule should be positioned in the perspective of sociodynamic reality, and the link with quality improvement could be a useful way to explain the complexity of actual acceptance and implementation. Change-related theories can be used for this purpose [2, 3].

In practice, the process of introduction of innovative technology is not as straightforward as Rogers presumes [1]. The theory of constructive technology assessment teaches us that technology innovations, when first introduced, not only shape the environment, but technology itself is influenced by sociodynamic and technical processes, thus resulting in a mutual influence on both the new technology and the actual environment in healthcare processes.

Constructive Technology Assessment (CTA) is an approach that starts from the paradigm of a dynamic relationship between (new) technology and environment. This can be embedded in the concept of a quality management system, both on the institutional and the process or project level. Both the basic features of the ISO-9002.4 guideline for quality systems and the Plan/Do/Check/Act cycle of Deming [4] can be used for this purpose. Thus a (preliminary) framework results that presents the innovation process as a diffusion, placed in the context of change and sociodymamic reality, whereas elements of quality management can be used to ensure an effective implementation process.

This framework has the following characteristics:

- The external macro diffusion process
- The internal embedding/diffusion on meso level

• Linking with the quality system on meso/micro level
• The internal innovation process on meso/micro level

THE CASE OF TELECONSULTATION IN
REHABILITATION MEDICINE

Teleconsultation in rehabilitation medicine will be presented as a case study. The first example reports a one-year pilot with teleconsultation on gait analysis using possibilities for video conferencing in combination with the mutual online availability of data on various movement-analysis procedures per patient. Second, the preliminary stages of tele-consultation between a rehabilitation hospital and free-standing (children's) physiotherapy practices will be presented. Using the above mentioned theory, an analysis can be made of the relevant aspects of such an introduction based on a study using constructive technology assessment.

Both innovations are mainly the result of "technology push" and typically are "external." Both practical and strategic factors contributed to the decision to implement them. As such, the various diffusion stages will be described, whereas the sociodynamic factors—again—seem to be extremely important. For the macro (regional) level, various scenarios were drawn to evaluate the actual development afterwards. When this is linked to the primary process using the steps of quality management, the improvement cycle is based both on quantitative indicators and sociodynamic feedback.

The complexity of teleconsultation is shown by dependence on technical features, minimally two organizations or organizational entities, the acceptances/applicability for the practicing professionals, and the value for the patient. In the case of gait analysis, high advantages for patients could be shown [5, 6], and costs were reduced. The consultant who was involved, however, felt that a less complex system would have been sufficient to achieve the same results (discontinuous video consultation). The case of teleconsultation with private practice (children's) physio-therapists was prepared by using CTA scenario techniques. Based on the four resulting scenarios, an evaluation of the actual implementation will be carried out. Both the scenarios and the progress of the implementation will be presented.

CONCLUSION

Quality management and innovation are closely related. Using relevant theories from both fields, the introduction of new technologies in health care can be analyzed and structured. Two cases of teleconsultation

Figure 11.1
Framework for Teleconsultation

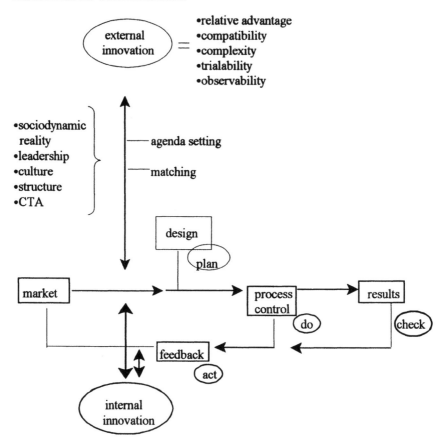

modalities in rehabilitation medicine are presented as examples (see Figure 11.1).

NOTES

[1] Rogers, E. M., *Diffusion of Innovations* (New York: Free Press, 1983).

[2] Pettigrew, A., and R. Whipp, *Managing Change for Competitive Success* (Oxford: Blackwell, 1991).

[3] Vinkenburg, H.H.M., "Stimuleren tot perfectie, kritieke factoren bij het verbeteren van dienstverlening," Academische thesis, Groningen, 1995.

[4] Deming, W. E., *Out of the Crisis* (New York: Cambridge University Press, 1982).

[5] Bloo, H.K.C., R.F.M. Kleissen, A. V. Nene, J. G. Becher, J. Harlaar, and G.

Zilvold, *Teleconsultation Using Movement Analysis Can Affect Patient Treatment* (Heidelberg: ESMAC, 1999).

[6] Bloo, H.K.C., E. Oosterhout-Mom, R.F.M. Kleissen, and J. Harlaar, "Teleconsultatie helpt bij het formuleren van behandelplannen," *Informatie & Zorg*, 29(2), 2000, 66–71.

Chapter 12

Empowering Nurses with Information Technology: The Challenge of Delivering Adequate Training

Laurence Alpay

INTRODUCTION

For the past few years there have been large investments in information technology (IT) in the health sector. However, at the same time there has been a lack of an equivalent investment in the education and training needed in this area [1]. One of the challenges in applying IT is in delivering adequate IT training. This is especially relevant to the nursing profession, which has generally derived less in benefits from existing IT training programs. This challenge raises some questions, for instance, about how to train better healthcare professionals to become IT skilled and knowledgeable and about how IT training programs will impact and affect changes in work practices in health care, particularly in improving information management.

This chapter is concerned with the issue of IT training for professional nurses in the context of a technologically evolving healthcare sector. The discussion draws from a recent empirical work involving practice nurses in primary care in the United Kingdom. The first part of the chapter reports on the use of IT by nurses and their obstacles to accessing IT training. Relevant findings from the empirical study are then described. The last two sections discuss a number of important aspects of IT training that are shared in hospitals and the community, and address the issue of IT training in the current context of the "transmural" redesign of care process. "Transmural care" is a fairly new concept in Dutch health care. It can be defined as patient-tailored care provided on the basis of close collaboration and joint responsibilities between hospitals and home care organizations. We use it here to reflect the cross-boundaries of IT training between primary and secondary care. The chapter largely refers to IT training of British nurses but also broadly examines this issue to encompass nurses everywhere.

USE OF INFORMATION TECHNOLOGY BY NURSES

Information technology is now essential to the development and delivery of health services. The increased usage of IT in health care has important implications for the way that all health professionals, including nurses, work [2]. Indeed, IT can support nurses in their daily activities such as retrieving medical records and recording assessment, planning, and interventions [3]. Additionally, the Internet and the World Wide Web give nurses the opportunity not only to access large volumes of information but also to communicate and collaborate with their peers worldwide [4, 5]. Furthermore, with the advent of the "new information age," computer-based collaborative work and communication are becoming relevant activities for all healthcare professionals [6].

However, while it is acknowledged that access to IT by nurses is important and beneficial [7], it is also widely recognized that nurses do not have adequate access to, and use of, IT [8]. In particular, recent work has suggested that a major challenge in the nurses' extended role is access to technology and the lack of appropriate skills. There is also some evidence that nurses do not always grasp the opportunity to enhance their practice and status with the introduction of IT in the workplace and to improve information management either within the hospital [9] or in primary care centers [10].

IT TRAINING FOR NURSES

IT usage also has important implications for the educational and training needs of all healthcare professionals (including nurses), to enable them to use the new technologies. Healthcare professionals are continuing to improve their computer literacy and to demonstrate a positive attitude toward computer use [11]. However, a substantial number of them have not yet acquired adequate knowledge of information technology and are in need of appropriate educational training in IT [12].

Providing proper IT training to nurses is difficult to achieve. Obstacles include inadequate (or nonexistent) training programs [13] and negative attitudes towards computer technologies [14]. In fact, when IT training programs exist, nurses are not always provided with IT educators who can appreciate their educational and learning needs. Thus, these instructors do not facilitate the teaching-learning process without provoking anxiety and discomfort [15, 16].

Other problems associated with IT training come from the nurses themselves, in that they may lack interest in and concern for IT and informatics. Many nurses in need of training in IT received their formal education before technology was integrated into the curriculum. Some of them have not been inclined to look into developing computer technologies [17]. Furthermore, for some, training in IT is only seen as relevant when the information content is deemed directly helpful, such as when linked with training in using specific information management systems.

Additionally, some nurses have difficulties in prioritizing their learning needs due to the large number of these needs including computerization and information technology [18]. Some nurses are being increasingly challenged with new educational demands (in order to use, for instance, clinical governance and evidence-based practice). Continuing education through open and distance learning is an attractive way to acquire informatics skills. However, these kinds of courses for newcomers to computers tend to expect their learners to be adaptable to novel modes of study.

Despite these problems, training healthcare professionals in IT, specifically practice nurses in primary care, is slowly evolving [16, 19]. In the United Kingdom, for instance, a number of initiatives have supported practice nurses in identifying their own training and development needs [20], and the Information for Health Strategy [21] has set out specific objectives to address these issues. At the international level, recent International Medical Informatics Association recommendations on education in health informatics [22] provide a framework for guiding development of training programs in informatics generally and IT in particular. Another well-known initiative has been the NIGHTINGALE project [23], which is dedicated to developing educational materials to train the nursing profession.

Alongside the obstacles reported above, one critical difficulty in developing adequate IT training is the lack of empirical evidence. This is especially salient in the case of practice nurses in primary care. Little is found in the literature on their current situation concerning IT training needs and requirements [4, 24, 25]. Examples of studies investigating IT training for general practice usually focused on general practitioners (GPs) rather than other members of the primary care team such as nurses [26].

EXAMPLE OF AN EMPIRICAL INVESTIGATION: THE PRACTIS PROJECT

The work reported here from the PRACTIS project (PRimary care nurses' Access to Communications Technology and Informatics Skills) has addressed the above issues for practice nurses in the United Kingdom. The aims of this project have been to provide empirical evidence on practice nurses' access to, and use of, IT in GP surgeries, together with their training needs in this area [27, 28].

Practice Nurses in Primary Care

Work practices for primary care nurses are evolving. The current trend in patient care delivery is toward integrated care, and primary care centers are organized around multiprofessional teams. Within the primary care team, the role of the nurse in the United Kingdom is changing rapidly. British nurses now play an active role in disease management and health promotion, while primary care groups (PCGs) [29] give nurses a clear role as part of PCG boards involved in commissioning health services for their local population.

These new developments have led to a burgeoning workload for the practice nurses, reflected in the way their numbers have increased in the United Kingdom by a huge 261 percent between 1988 and 1995 [13]. The current role of the practice nurse incorporates a need to be proficient in using information technology, which will enable them to access, manage, and disseminate the data that develops from all this increased activity.

Methods

Empirical data (quantitative and qualitative) were collected from practice nurses working in different GP practices in North, South, and Mid Buckinghamshire. The GP surgeries varied in size and location. A survey questionnaire was addressed to 225 practice nurses in Buckinghamshire. Four practice nurses, an in-house computer trainer and a healthcare development specialist from the Buckinghamshire Health Authority were consulted for advice and piloting the questionnaire. The questionnaire was in four parts to cover details of the nurses and their surgeries, their access to IT, their use of IT, and their training needs. The questionnaire included some open questions and space for comments. Responses (57%) were received from the different types of practices.

Issues emerging from the results of the questionnaire were explored in two focus groups. The focus groups were comprised of 12 practice nurses. Various issues addressed in the focus groups, including those related to IT training, focused on the nurses' training needs for IT and their use of IT for educational purposes. Each focus group of six nurses, representative of the survey, lasted approximately 90 minutes.

Relevant Results

Several kinds of methods of training were reported.
Colleague's Help: The most common method was to learn from watch-

ing a colleague and then to have hands-on experience, often using a trial-and-error method. Although 43 percent of the sample (N = 51) found this method adequate, this was not seen as an ideal method. Mistakes can be perpetrated and go uncorrected for considerable lengths of time, and easier ways of using the technology remain undiscovered.

In-house Trainer: The nurses thought it would help to have a knowledgeable person on site to whom they could go for help. However, in the current situation, 51 percent reported that an in-house trainer was simply not available (N = 61).

External Trainer: A large majority of nurses (90%) reported that external trainers were usually not available (N = 108). However, outside trainers were sometimes used when a new system was installed.

User Manual and Help on Screen: The nurses suggested that a user-friendly manual would be useful. It was also felt that it would be helpful to write things down oneself in a way that could be understood. A surprising 80 percent reported that there was no computer manual at hand (N = 95). Alongside a paper-based manual, help on screen was also not available for 62 percent of the nurses (N = 74).

Types of IT Training

The nurses wanted to have initial basic training on computers and also on the specific systems they used. When the nurses were asked about their initial IT training, it seems that those who received it were trained on two specific software systems (i.e., EMIS and Meditel specifically developed for use in GP surgeries). Being knowledgeable about only a couple of specific systems is a limitation for the nurses. Overall, nurses were found to lack an overview of what IT can and cannot do. Training in basic IT skills appeared to be minimal, as less than 5 percent of the nurses had received training in using any of the categories investigated, which included word processing, CD-ROM, e-mail, and the Internet.

Barriers to IT Training

Ideally, the nurses would like time for designated training in IT. Furthermore, delay in obtaining training is also an issue. One nurse reported that although further training has been promised, it was going to take months to get it. As well as the time factor, lack of funding available to support IT training creates a difficult situation for the nurses.

Attitudes regarding the use of IT are closely intertwined with the training received. Although nurses were generally motivated to use IT, problems of attitude remain toward computerization. For example, half of the nurses did not feel at ease about using the surgery computer systems and two-thirds of the nurses who used e-mail and the Internet said they lacked confidence.

TOWARD A "TRANSMURAL" APPROACH TO IT TRAINING

The PRACTIS project has brought new empirical evidence on the difficulties with and subsequent needs of IT training for practice nurses in primary care. Even though the study in PRACTIS was limited by its geographical context, the situation of British practice nurses is not unique, and findings from the PRACTIS project can offer useful insights to other primary care centers. Practice nurses in other parts of Europe are also facing difficulties with their access to, use of, and professional development in information technology. In the Netherlands, for instance, these kinds of problems have been reported [30] and experiments to address these issues are being undertaken [31].

The problems of providing adequate IT training are also shared across the various points of care, both in hospitals and in the community. Within the context of shared and transmural care, such as between primary and secondary care, results from the empirical work (such as in PRACTIS) should be of benefit to all the sectors of health care. While the actual contents of IT training targeted to nurses will (or may) vary between GP practices and hospitals, there are a number of important aspects related to IT training that are of consideration in both healthcare sectors. These issues, discussed below, can be viewed as "transmural" in the development of IT training programs for nurses in the primary and the secondary care sectors.

Facilitating Technological Changes and Integration within the Organization

IT training can act as a facilitator for the integration of technological changes within the organization. Healthcare professionals need to learn IT skills that can help them, for instance, reduce difficulties of IT access and use and manage electronic information. Managing information is an important activity of nursing care, and IT training can help nurses with this task. The nurses interviewed in PRACTIS had to work with different practices for recording information, and problems with managing the information occur when people use different codes to record the same types of information. Additionally, nurses in PRACTIS had to handle an overload of work brought by computer use. The duplication of effort occurred quite frequently because of the way information was generally managed. IT training can also help nurses to manage technical problems they encounter. For example, nurses reported that there are problems with access to passwords, both within and between surgeries. This took up time that could be spent more effectively. Coupled with that, there was not always someone available who could help the nurse with this or with other information she needed to know in order to access and use the computer.

Sharing of Knowledge and Expertise

IT training can empower healthcare professionals with the necessary skills to develop and use a global network of knowledge and expertise within their own speciality, like nursing. The nurses interviewed in PRACTIS were interested in developing a computerized network to exchange information and to disseminate specialist skills (as in the GP-UK for instance [32]) but did not have the training and support to enable them to set this up between the surgeries. This aspect is closely related to the issue of nursing intelligence, that is, information gathered from nurses in their nursing work and the nurses' role in utilizing such intelligence [33]. Capitalizing on nursing intelligence is increasingly becoming a priority for nurses, as recently illustrated by Ballard [34].

Moreover, the nurses were very aware of the benefits of having an Intranet computer network within the surgery, although few of them were actually able to use one. They mentioned how it would save time by giving access to patient notes in more than one location at once. They also saw benefits in being able to communicate with doctors and receptionists via internal e-mail to elicit a quick response without having to interrupt a consultation.

Supporting Culture's Change

The introduction of information technology in the workplace not only has an impact on changes in work practices but also on other related aspects, such as changes in roles and responsibilities and changes in "culture." For example, roles and responsibilities of healthcare professionals, including nurses, have been reported to change in relation to electronic access and data entry of patient information [35]. It is recognized that a culture change in nursing is happening: information technology is seen by some nurses and nurse leaders to support rather than conflict with activities [36]. However, such a change seems difficult to achieve in the short term when computer resistance and computer anxiety still affect a large number of nurses [15].

In some cases within the culture of GP practices, the need for nurses to have access to computers and to have adequate training does not have a high priority. GPs often expect practice nurses when presented with a new computer system to be able to know how to use the computer even though they may have no previous experience of that system [37]. It would seem that GPs and administrative staff have other needs and uses for IT and often are not aware of how the nurses could use and access electronic information and may feel that nurses might not have the confidence and ability to use IT.

Our analysis from focus groups in PRACTIS suggested that GPs vary considerably in the way they prioritize nurses' training needs and in their perception of the practice nurse role. This observation is also relevant to the perceptions of surgery administrative staff, who do not always understand why nurses need to record certain information. Thus the nurses' access to and use of computers in the surgery is highly dependent on the attitude and understanding of IT of others working within the surgery [35]. Where there is a consensus and competence in using IT, results are very helpful for collaborative integrated practice. There is still a huge unrealized potential to improve overall conditions in the working environment with the efficient use of IT, and a need to involve nursing staff in the specifications and implementation of IT services.

Supporting Professional Development and Proactivity

Culture change for nurses also relates to their professional development and proactivity. Older nurses usually feel that they are of a generation that received no opportunity to use computers during their formal education. The nurses were very aware that they could use IT skills to access knowledge and develop new learning for their continuing professional development. For example, the nurses wanted to be able to communicate with colleagues, manage information, educate themselves and their patients, and save themselves time by better understanding how to access and use IT. The nurses expressed a desire to understand basic IT skills and management of information and not just to be able to use software already in place in the surgery.

Nurses tend to work within a computer environment that can deal with the complexities of the care they plan and deliver rather than working with computer technologies that require them to adapt their practices to the computer environment. One way to do so is for nurses to be more proactive in seeking out how IT, coupled with adequate information management, will improve their practice [38]. The view that nurses ought to be involved in the IT revolution is also echoed by Negron [15] and Keen and Malby [9]. It is through models like the one proposed by Nagelkerk et al. [16] that nurses can prepare themselves for computerization, and change their negative attitudes. Those authors identified six factors that will successfully help nurses in nursing informatics, including strong leadership, effective communication, and organized training sessions. Furthermore, in order to be more proactive, nurses need to be reflective. For example, nurses should assess and aim to raise their levels of concerns in their use and access of IT [19].

IT TRAINING IN THE CONTEXT OF CARE PROCESS REDESIGN

The integration of IT in the care process brings a need to evaluate, analyze, and eventually redesign the chain of care in order to better serve strategic objectives and performance goals. One approach, such as business process redesign (BPR), is already being successfully applied in health care to achieve this aim [39]. Examples from the literature provide interesting insights into the advantages and potential pitfalls of this redesign activity, for example, in hospitals, as in the case of cardiovascular surgery [40] and laboratory services [41].

In the context of ongoing developments in reshaping care process, providing the appropriate IT training to healthcare professionals, including nurses, will be a relevant factor to the successful outcomes of this redesign task. Reengineering of care process includes the need to examine the tasks people do, and how well trained they are to do them when they have to use information- and communication-based technologies. It is clear from our empirical study that there is a need for more than just giving technical training and support to the nurses, although this is very important. Indeed, there is a cultural as well as an organizational problem of integrating the use of IT into working practice in primary care. Roles, responsibilities, and relationships are changing through the assertion of IT within the workplace. This translates into a need for effective management of information, which can be achieved where there is ease of use and understanding of the capabilities of IT.

The implications of work redesign and reengineering for nurses (especially nurse executives) have been recognized [42], and models have been proposed [43, 44]. Becoming knowledgeable in IT and its potential and keeping well informed of new developments are some of the most important ones. Such tools as the MMT (management of medical technology) proposed by Geisler [45], for example, provide a useful framework to achieve this professional development. Furthermore, alongside the need to understand informatics, related skills such as human relations and business processes are increasingly being given consideration [12].

The nature of new IT training programs, as well as the effects these will have on care process redesign, needs to be investigated further. One approach is to take a sociotechnical view [46], as illustrated for nursing administration by Happ [47]. In this approach, the investigation focuses on how both the sociological and the technological environments of workers (e.g., nurses) are an integral part of all aspects of their working practice. For example, one can examine how nursing information management is best performed and applied through the use of information and communication technologies. Tools to address this issue have already been proposed [48]. Moreover, through a sociotechnical approach, interactions between the users of the technology (e.g., the nurses) and the technology itself are researched. The end objective is a joint optimization of the technical and social systems [49].

Another research orientation is in cognitive science, which seeks to promote the "usability" and "learnability" of IT in the realm of human-computer interaction within the workplace [50]. Cognitive science can be used to inform designers of technology for GP surgeries or hospital wards to enable IT to be used more easily and effectively. If optimal use is to be made of the opportunities presented by the use of IT, then an understanding of the interactions and relationships between users of the technology needs to be gained. For the nursing profession, work in cognitive science, coupled with research in human-computer interactions, will help in developing a work environment where computer use is integrated in nursing care, meets ergonomics requirements, and supports various human interactions and communications [51].

CONCLUSION

The role IT training has to play for professional nurses in the climax of reengineering of healthcare processes should not be underestimated. Nurses form a separate professional body and, as viewed by some [52], nursing informatics is becoming a distinctive discipline from medical informatics. Thus, nurses have distinct work requirements, including the need for dedicated IT training programs. For nurses to be part of the major transformations occurring in the delivery of care, effort must take place to provide easy access to IT training as well as to improve the quality of that training. Through their reorganizational changes, it is the responsibilities of the requisite institutions to ensure that nurses (involved at all levels of nursing care and management) are given the opportunities to acquire the necessary IT skills. The increasing role of the informatics nurse specialist, for example [53], can support the organization in creating these opportunities.

As expected, individual institutions may not always have the resources to achieve this goal alone. Indeed, healthcare administrators have had to contain their expenditures while at the same time improve both the quality and quantity of educational provision. It is through joint efforts that collaborative initiatives in developing IT training for nurses (and other healthcare professionals) can yield tangible benefits for all parties.

Alongside joint collaborations, there is also the need to encourage more empirical investigations into IT use in hospitals and in GP practices. It is important to examine not only nurses' IT skills but also their understanding of information management using those skills. Investigating the situation of IT training and professional development for healthcare professionals will further our understanding of their needs and help to prepare the necessary actions. It will also empower healthcare professionals, including nurses, to become better equipped to meet the technological advances of the coming years with confidence.

ACKNOWLEDGMENTS

Thanks to Angela Russell (The Open University, United Kingdom) for her invaluable contribution to the PRACTIS project and for her feedback on this manuscript. Thanks also to Cees Zeelenberg and Gerard Freriks (TNO-PG, The Netherlands), and William Goossen (ACQUEST, The Netherlands) for their comments.

NOTES

[1] Norris, A., and J. Brittain, "Education, Training and the Development of Healthcare Informatics," *Health Informatics Journal*, 6(4), 2000, 189–195.

[2] Alpay, L., G. Needham, and P. Murray, "The Potential of Information Technology for Nurses in Primary Care: A Review of Issues and Trends," *Primary Health Care Research and Development*, 1(1), 2000, 5–13.

[3] Ronald, J., "The Computer as a Partner in Nursing Practice: Implications for Curriculum Change," *Lecture Notes in Medical Informatics*, 46, 1991, 149–153.

[4] Murray, P., "Research and the Internet: Some Practical and Ethical Issues," *Nursing Online*, 10(28), 1996, 12–16.

[5] Murray, P., and D. Anthony, "Current and Future Models for Nursing e-journals: Making the Most of the Web's Potential," *International Journal of Medical Informatics*, 1998.

[6] Alpay, L., and H. Heathfield, "A Review of Telematics in Healthcare: Evolution, Challenges and Caveats," *Health Informatics Journal*, 3(2), 1997, 81–92.

[7] Moritz, P., "Information Technology—A Priority for Nursing Research," *Computers in Nursing*, 8(3), 1990, 111–115.

[8] Hasman, A., "Education and Training in Health Informatics," *Computer Methods and Programs in Biomedicine*, 45, 1994, 41–43.

[9] Keen, J., and R. Malby, "Nursing Power and Practice in the United Kingdom National Health Service," *Journal of Advanced Nursing*, 17, 1992, 863–870.

[10] Carlile, S., and A. Sefton, "Healthcare and the Information Age: Implications for Medical Education," *Medical Journal of Australia*, 168(7), 1998, 340–343.

[11] Scarpa, R., S. Smeltzer, and B. Jasion, "Attitudes of Nurses Toward Computerization: A Replication," *Computers in Nursing*, 10(2), 1992, 72–80.

[12] Staggers, N., C. Gassert, and D. Skiba, "Health Professionals' Views on Informatics Education," *JAMIA*, 7(6), 2000, 550–558.

[13] Miller, A., and R. Jeffcote, "Practice Nurses and Computing: Some Evidence on Utilization, Training and Attitudes to Computer Use," *Health Informatics Journal*, 3, 1997, 10–16.

[14] Lacey, D., "Nurses' Attitudes Towards Computerization: A Review of the Literature," *Journal of Nursing Management*, 1, 1993, 239–243.

[15] Negron, J., "The Impact of Computer Anxiety and Computer Resistance on the Use of Computer Technology by Nurses," *Journal of Nursing Staff Development*, 11(3), 1995, 172–175.

[16] Nagelkerk, L., P. Ritola, and P. Vandort, "Nursing Informatics: The Trend of the Future," *Journal of Continuing Education in Nursing*, 29(1), 1998, 17–21.

[17] Roberts, J., and V. Peel, "Getting IT into Shape—External Factors Effecting the Potential Benefits from Health Informatics," in Pappas, M. et al. (Eds.), *Proceedings of Medical Informatics Europe (MIE '97)* (Amsterdam: IOS Press, 1997), pp. 825–828.

[18] Lindner, R., "A Framework to Identify Learning Needs for Continuing Nurse Education Using Information Technology," *Journal of Advanced Nursing*, 27, 1998, 1017–1020.

[19] Barnett, D., "Informing the Nursing Professions with IT," in Greenes, A., M. Peterson, and L. Protti (Eds.), *Proceedings of the 8th World Congress on Medical Informatics (MEDINFO '95)* (Amsterdam: North-Holland, 1995), pp. 1316–1320.

[20] NHSTD, *Education and Training Program in IM&T for Clinicians: A Framework for Nurses* (Bristol: NHSTD Publications, 1995).

[21] DoH—Department of Health, *Information for Health—An Information Strategy for the Modern NHS 1998–2005* (London: NHS Executive Publications, 1998).

[22] IMIA-WG1, "The IMIA Curriculum Guidelines for Health and Medical Informatics," *Methods of Information in Medicine*, 39, 2000, 204–277.

[23] Mantas, J., "Nursing Informatics Educational Issues: The NIGHTINGALE Project," in Brender, M., B. Christensen, M. Scherrer, and G. McNair (Eds.), *Proceedings of Medical Informatics Europe '96* (Amsterdam: IOS Press, 1996), pp. 804–807.

[24] Wright, G., "A Review of Current IM&T Provision Within Pre- and Post-registration Nurse Training," in *Health Services Management Unit Center for Health Informatics* (Manchester: University of Manchester Publications, 1994).

[25] Simpson, G., and M. Kenrick, "Nurses' Attitudes Towards Computerization in Clinical Practice in a British General Hospital," *Computers in Nursing*, 15(1), 1997, 37–42.

[26] Ahmed, A., and A. Berlin, "Information Technology in General Practice: Current Use and View on Future Development," *Journal of Informatics in Primary Care*, November 1997.

[27] Russell, A., and L. Alpay, "Practice Nurses' Training in Information Technology: Report on an Empirical Investigation," *Health Informatics Journal*, 6(3), 2000, 142–146.

[28] Alpay, L., and A. Russell (in press), "Information Technology Training in Primary Care: The Nurses' Voice," submitted to *Computers in Nursing*.

[29] DoH—Department of Health, *The New NHS—Modern and Dependable* (London: NHS Executive Publications, 1997).

[30] Goossen, W., "Overview of Health Care and Nursing Informatics in the Netherlands," *Health Informatics*, 2(1), 1996, 9–20.

[31] Welling, N., and D. Delnoij, "The Practice Nurse in British Family Practice. Lessons for Dutch Experiments," *Verpleegkunde*, 12(30), 1997, 131–139.

[32] Thomas, R., and S. James, "Informal Communications Networking Among Health Professionals: A Study of GP-UK," *Health Informatics Journal*, 5(2), 1999, 74–81.

[33] Ballard, E., "Important Considerations about Nursing Intelligence and Information Systems," in Gerdin, L., N. Talberg, and J. Wainright (Eds.), *Nursing Informatics—The Impact of Nursing Knowledge on Health Care Informatics* (Amsterdam: IOS Press, 1997), pp. 44–49.

[34] Ballard, E., "Nursing Information for Electronic Clinical Exchange (NIECE)," *Health Informatics Journal*, 5, 1999, 3–8.

[35] Herbert, M., "Impact of IT on Health Care Professionals: Changes in Work and the Productivity Paradox," *Health Services Management Research*, 11, 1998, 69–79.

[36] Procter, P., "Responses Within the Virtual Conference, Action One: Culture Change," *Proceedings of the Second National Conference of the CTI Center for Nursing and Midwifery* (Sheffield: CTINM Publications, 1998).

[37] Lock, K., "Primary Health Care: Using Computer to Enhance Care in a GP Practice," *Nursing Times*, 91(18), 1995, 36–38.

[38] Marin, H., I. Cunha, and C. Safran, "Nurses' Requirements for Information Technology in the Next Millennium," in Cesnik, B., C. McCray, and M. Scherrer (Eds.), *Proceedings of the 9th World Congress on Medical Informatics (MEDINFO '98)* (Amsterdam: IOS Press, 1998), pp. 1314–1317.

[39] Strong, A., and H. Yarde, "Achieving Outcomes through Organizational Redesign," *Nursing Clinic of North America*, 32(3), 1997, 603–614.

[40] Tunick, P., S. Etkin, A. Horrocks, G. Jeglinski, J. Kelly, and P. Sutton, "Reengineering a Cardiovascular Surgery Service," *Joint Commission Journal on Quality Improvement*, 23(4), 1997, 203–216.

[41] Kelly, D., "Reframing Beliefs about Work and Change Processes in Redesigning Laboratory Services," *Joint Commission Journal on Quality Improvement*, 24(23), 1998, 154–167.

[42] Cabtree Tonges, M. (1993), "Reengineering The Work Redesign—Technology Link," *JONA*, 23(10), 1993, 15–22.

[43] Gassert, C. (1990), "Structured Analysis: Methodology for Developing a Model for Defining Nursing Information Systems Requirements," *Advances in Nursing Science*, 13(2), 1990, 53–62.

[44] Currel, R. (1992), "Models for Nursing—The Paradox of Business Activity Modelling," in Lun, P. et al. (Eds.), *Proceedings of MEDINFO 92* (Amsterdam: Elsevier Science Publishers BV/IMIA, 1992), pp. 964–969.

[45] Geisler, E. (2000), "Medical Doctor, Organizational Doctor and Technical Doctor; Management of Medical Technology (MTT) and the Revolution in Modern Health Care Delivery," *International Journal of Healthcare Technology and Management*, 2, 2000, 1–14.

[46] Berg, M. (1999), "Patient Care Information Systems and Health Care Work: A Socio-technical Approach," *International Journal of Medical Informatics*, 55, 1999, 87–101.

[47] Happ, M. (1993), "Sociotechnical System Theory: Analysis and Applications

for Nursing Administration," *Journal of Nursing Administration*, 23(6), 1993, 47–54.

[48] Goossen, W. (2000) *Towards Strategic Use of Nursing Information in the Netherlands* (Groningen: Rijkuniversiteit [proefschrift], 2000).

[49] Herbst, P. (1976) *Sociotechnical Design: Strategies in Multidisciplinary Research* (London: Tavistock Publications, 1976).

[50] Patel, V., A. Kushniruk, S. Yang, and J-F. Yale (2000), "Impact of a Computer-based Patient Record System on Data Collection, Knowledge Organisation and Reasoning," *JAMIA*, 7(6), 2000, 569–585.

[51] Goossen, W. (in press), "Human Interaction," in Mantas, J. (Ed.), *Nursing Informatics of the Nightingale Project*.

[52] Masys, D., P. Brennan, J. Ozbolt, M. Corn, and E. Shortliffe (2000), "Are Medical and Nursing Informatics Distinct Disciplines? The 1999 ACMI Debate," *JAMIA*, 7(3), 2000, 304–312.

[53] Lange, L. (1997), "Informatics Nurse Specialist: Roles in Healthcare Organisations," *Nursing Administrative Quality*, 21(3), 1997, 1–10.

Chapter 13

Careful Hospital Design: The Act of Balancing Stakeholder Interests

Rennee Dooyeweerd and Roel W. Schuring

INTRODUCTION

The nature of a hospital building determines to a certain extent the effectiveness of healthcare (and other) processes that take place in that building. As Winston Churchill said, "First we shape our buildings, thereafter they shape us" [1]. This is certainly true of the hospital building where the organizational functioning and the efficiency of its structuring depend (among other factors) on space, distance, location, and other building structure–related dimensions. The underlying belief is that designing hospital infrastructure is an organizational question. By this, we mean that the physical building structure is or should be the (literally) concrete reflection of the organizational design as well as that the organization is partly shaped, certainly influenced, supported, or hampered by its physical delineation (or armor). A careful hospital design supports the processes that have to take place within the building to treat patients in an effective and efficient manner.

How do we realize this? The way this problem was coped with up to now was mostly by building on past experiences. If needed, concepts that have proven satisfactory in other situations were modified. The choices of design (and their possible motivation) were made in a "wicked" process in which an architect's tacit knowledge (based on training and his/her own former experiences) played a prominent role. In many building projects, relevant stakeholders in the hospital were consulted through numerous user groups, using various design techniques. This led to adjustments to the existing concepts rather than innovative new designs. We want to stress that hospital design has indeed changed over the years. The central hall with all the patients in the "Hospital de Paris" was incomparable to the pavilion structure that we found in Barcelona or the Breitfuss model that we see in Germany.

Nevertheless, hospital design is still a quest for the Holy Grail. This has to do with the ever-continuing change in the field, including changes in patterns of morbidity, advances in medical technology, changing demands and opinions, and new management insights. We presume, however, that the problem is not only due to these changes and bears a more fundamental nature.

In order to be effective, a building structure should facilitate individual doctors in performing their various activities. But at the same time, it must not complicate the indispensable cooperation and communication between specialists and multidisciplinary diagnosis and treatment of patients. Structure must contribute to efficiency and transparency of processes involving different patient categories, but without fragmenting the work processes of doctors too much and decentralizing technology to an unmanageable scale. We presume that this will never be achieved, as long as a single ordering principle in the design process is used.

The quest for the grail continues as some new hospital building projects come up with new concepts. Again, more patient focus and better use of resources is claimed. However, we propose a new approach to the problem. Our approach is to retain the focus on the processes in the organization during the design of hospitals. We presume that it is possible to balance the support for all these processes by balancing the process requirements of the various stakeholders. Stakeholders are interested in the role that a hospital building plays in relation to their own work. At the same time, stakeholders in a hospital are mutually dependent. The contribution of any of them is instrumental to the organization as a whole, and thus, to each other.

As a starting point for design, the interdependence and the varying interests of stakeholders should be identified. We propose a "balanced scorecard" approach balancing stakeholder interests, in order to fulfill a prerequisite for optimally attaining the ultimate goal of satisfying the interest of the patient.

This chapter is an exploration of the field that ends with a preliminary draft of a "balanced scorecard" approach of stakeholder interests for careful hospital design. To end with that prototype, we will first discuss the topic of organizational design for hospital processes in general. This will further illustrate the complex nature of this design. Subsequently, we will discuss the nature of performance on an operational level and the stakeholder theory. In the final version of our approach we want to include the interests of stakeholders inside and outside the boundaries of the hospital. Also, it needs to consider the upcoming changes in the environment. The instrument that we are going to generate does not restrict hospital design to a single shape. It is merely an instrument to assess various designs.

ORGANIZATIONAL DESIGN FOR HOSPITAL PROCESSES: AN OVERVIEW

The starting point to the approach that we want to generate lies in the focus on *processes* in organizations. Among other contributions, a number of lines of thought are relevant. First, designing a building that can contribute to the performance of a hospital organization touches different streams of literature but is evidently related to the problem of organizational design as it is dealt with in operations management. In this light, a hospital is nothing more than a complex "production" system: a healthcare delivery system. From this operations management field, various techniques can be used, such as group technology [2] and systematic layout planning [3]. Both techniques consider multiple criteria in the process of optimization of the structure. Group technology brings together groups of tasks on the basis of logistics and functions, while systematic layout planning minimizes distances after determining the relevance of closeness. Still, optimization is difficult in hospitals when these techniques are being used. A hospital has to perform several functions (consulting, diagnosing, treating, research, teaching) and is accordingly comprised of various processes that together can be labeled the set of primary processes. Each process places its own demands on the functional closeness, distance, and process order. These instruments are valuable to hospital design but are not a definitive key in the quest for the grail. This conclusion also applies to similar instruments that are more specific to hospital design [4, 5].

The value of these instruments may grow once we no longer take the existing care processes in an organization for granted but on the contrary try to reshape our processes. This area of business process redesign [6] has been applied in health care successfully [7]. Restructured processes provide a clearer basis for optimizing the layout of an organization. The complement to business process redesign (BPR) is improvement of processes [8, 9]. In this field there is still a long way to go in health care [10]. Again, a clearer structure provides a basis for optimizing the layout.

If we have different contingencies or organizational technologies, we might end up with different processes and thus with different organizational structures. Remember, our point of view is that the physical building structure is or should be the (literally) concrete reflection of the organizational design as well as that the organization is partly shaped, certainly influenced, supported, or hampered by its physical delineation (or armor). That is why this approach is crucial to our study. The central argument is that the effectiveness and efficiency of the organization are determined by both the consistency of the system with the environment in which it operates (external fit) and the fit of the elements of the configuration itself (internal fit) [11].

Donaldson [12] reviewed the critics on contingency approaches that link the organizational structure to size of the organization, complexity of the work processes, degree of routine, age, stability of the environment, and other characteristics. He concluded that contingency theory can be defended. We faintly recognize this when hospital designs are based on some sort of categorization of patients as a first ordering principle or primary design parameter for the organization and its processes. Depending on the primary order chosen, a different physical building structure will arise. "Organizing around patients" has known a lot of varieties.

A few basic ordering principles can be used as a primary design parameter for the hospital structure, depending partly on the scale of the hospital (based on [5]):

- Patient categories: bundling facilities for a certain group of patients
- Length of patients' stay: separate clinical, ambulatory and day treatment units
- Professional groups: separation of nursing and medical units
- Medical specialists
- Surgical/nonsurgical specialists
- Individual medical specialists
- Related or corresponding medical specialists: clusters of specialists
- Geographically: separation of basic or day-to-day care and high-level care

The problem remains that there is no definite starting point. None of these principles has proven to be of lasting value. As a consequence, the organizational and building design of hospitals is still oscillating between different extremes in which medical specialists and groups of facilities or departments are the major entities by which to categorize patients. It is difficult to believe that future attempts to find the "final answer" by continuing this process of oscillation will succeed.

This also leads to different archetypes of hospital buildings. The early hospitals were designed around groups of patients treated within the different medical specialities. This "vertical differentiation"[13] of hospital care, leading to the specialist-oriented building archetype, was suitable (and still suffices) in cases in which patients are treated by specialists very individually. With the increasing specialization (and accordingly the number of specialities) and the advances of medical technology that have driven hospital care into a broad variety of treatments, the organization and its delivery processes, when this "ordering by specialty" is followed persistently, become very fragmented and inefficient in utilizing resources [14]. This so-called specialists model is currently still prominently visible in the building structure of some academic hospitals.

Most hospital buildings currently in use in the Netherlands are designed around distinctively different functions. They are built up of a nursing block, an ambulatory care facility, and a diagnostic research and treatment section, reflecting (sometimes even recognizable from the outside) the division into mainstreams or product lines of clinical and ambulatory care [15]. Within these building blocks, a division into (groups of) medical specialties is commonly found. Over the last decade a unit for day treatment was often established, which is on the border between clinical and ambulatory care. In terms of processes, most of the individual care processes (in which a crucial choice is whether hospital admission is necessary or not) are concentrated in one or two parts of the hospital and relatively efficient. The coordination around patients who are admitted, going "across product lines," is critical. The work processes, especially for medical professionals, are divided into two physically separate parts of the hospital in this so-called services model.

Recently, a trend is showing that hospitals developing new plans are shifting to "new" patient-oriented and process-based arrangements in which facilities, staff, and doctors (for part of their work) are ordered around processes for different (sufficiently large and homogeneous) groups of patients [5]. The patient orientation is not so new (actually it was envisioned and advocated as early as the early 1970s) [14], but now the renewed "all encompassing" perspective on primary processes is translated into physical clustering of facilities around patient groups with related complaints. Special attention is given more and more to organizing for multidisciplinary care and therefore a part of the activities are grouped into multidisciplinary medical units in which doctors work all or part of their time. Central to this approach is the idea that the "doctor comes to the patient," and not vice versa. The formulated objectives are shorter throughput times, efficiency, and effectiveness for the individual patients. But doctors are, and will want to stay, involved in several patient categories and need to stay in touch with colleagues from their own and related disciplines. Strict compliance with patient-oriented structuring of the hospital will complicate or restrain this.

The way the complex dilemma of finding a hospital design has been handled up to now is usually by building on past experiences and adopting—and where necessary modifying—concepts that have proven satisfactory in other situations. The choices of design that are made and their motivation, which is often not made explicit, are the results of a serendipitous, "wicked" process [16]. The architect uses mostly forms of tacit knowledge to come to solve the design problem. This knowledge is based on the architect's training and education, along with experience, which builds on former projects. To find a suitable hospital design, one has to satisfy the needs of all relevant parties in the situation at hand. Therefore, in current design practice in most hospital development projects, many of the users are consulted, through numerous user groups, using different techniques. However, this often leads to situational adjustments to the existing concepts rather than innovative new designs. Often it also does not provide clear, rational arguments why the traditional design solutions are chosen. In our view, to argue the choice of any design solution, a structural analysis of performance aspects, followed by an explicit judgment of design solutions according to these performances, would be desired but all too often is not found.

Our conclusion is that process orientation has been a dominant factor for hospital design in the past. This makes sense indeed, as hospitals are there to *work*, like any other organization has to work.

COMPLICATIONS IN PROCESS-ORIENTED DESIGN OF HOSPITALS

There are a number of complicating factors in the process-oriented design of hospitals. One is the continuing change in technology and values. To illustrate this, a short historical overview shows that hospital management's primary emphasis in the Netherlands first shifted from caring for patients to more professionally nursing patients in the 1960s [17]. Development of a lot of diagnostic and therapeutic methods shifted the emphasis to providing facilities and services to the medical professionals in a functional divisionalized structure [18] in the 1970s. The early 1980s showed increasing attention to providing service to the different streams of clinical and ambulatory patients (to prevent and/or compensate for the existing waiting lists) in a structure divisionalized corresponding to these mainstreams. After 1985 the governmental budgeting system shifted the management focus and made medical diagnosis and treatment the primary process of hospitals, which evolved into a professional bureaucracy operating within externally imposed tight budgets. The 1990s brought back the attention to caring for patients, but in a much more encompassing manner than before and in terms of "appropriate" or "sized to fit" care (*Zorg op Maat*). This illustrates only a fraction of the changes in technology and society that a process-oriented hospital design should take into account.

Another complicating factor is the hybrid nature of the processes in the organization. Woodward [19] faced this problem when setting up her renowned typology and simply focused on industries in her dataset with a nonhybrid character. Hospitals, as we know them by now, inevitably are a mixture of technologies and processes. The contingency propositions for the design of an organization can sometimes be contradictory, and a balance of design propositions has to be found to obtain an internal or design parameter fit that leads to higher performance [20]. The hospital design has to facilitate individual doctors in performing their various activities. At the same time the division of work must not complicate the indispensable cooperation and communication between specialties and multidisciplinary diagnosis and treatment of patients. Structure must also contribute to efficiency and transparency of processes involving different patient categories. On the other hand, it may not fragment the work processes of doctors too much, and allocating the technology to processes may not lead to decentralization of technology to a scale that leads to inefficient use and is impossible to manage. The layout must support efficient and mostly separate transportation of patients, information, and all kinds of goods, but this might lead to unavoidable compromises to the chosen primary ordering principle. Evolving medical possibilities, increasing specialization, and the pressure for more customer-oriented healthcare services just adds to the complexity of the problem noted. As a consequence, the organizational structure is of Mintzberg's different ideal types or a "hybrid" [18]. But what does this mean to the building design?

A final complicating factor is that the requirements of processes depend on the stakeholder that is being asked. Hospital design is essentially about finding a configuration that can meet the numerous requirements and demands placed on it by many. The hospital design should enable and find a compromise between the necessary involvement and interaction of hospital constituents as actors in different processes, the operational cohesion within the primary processes, and the functional cohesion in terms of grouping and locating resources (facilities) into units of a manageable scale [21, 22]. The contribution of the physical surroundings to effective and efficient processes is, of course, one of many influences and hard to determine to its fullest extent. But a suitable building structure certainly is, even in a most limited view, a prerequisite and should be instrumental to the organization and its constituents. If the building structure does not comply with the processes that are to be executed, it will be hard if not impossible to organize around it and run the processes efficiently in despite of it.

In our attempt to find an approach to process-oriented design of hospitals, we propose a more prominent role for the process interest of stakeholders in the organization. Stakeholders can be the link between contingencies and organizational design, as they have a boundary-spanning role in the various contingencies. Also, the process interest of stakeholders nicely covers the diversity and complexity of processes in the organization. Stakeholders are the explorers of developments in the environment and can help to create a hospital design that is fit for the future. Finally, stakeholder orientation can help to focus on the patients' interest, as we have substantiated before.

On the basis of this, a structural analysis of performance aspects should be possible. This will not lead to one best structure under given conditions. There might be equifinality, which means that multiple organizational forms can be equally effective [23]. Any structure may have many functions and any function may be fulfilled by alternative structures or processes [24], which means different (production) systems can lead to the same level of performance, or vice versa, the same structures can perform differently [25, 26].

Finally, the design process is not straightforward but rather a complex, interactive process in which a lot of relevant parties (stakeholders) are involved and influence the choice of organizational design [27, 28]. The solution that will be chosen is the one estimated or perceived to attain the highest performance within the given context or contingencies. But what this performance constitutes may not always be unambiguous. The parties that are involved in this choice, the stakeholders, will have different perceptions of what constitutes performance, which is thus multivariable. We will further discuss this in the next section on performance.

OUR CONSTRUCT OF PERFORMANCE

To operationalize the concept of performance for hospital design we will first argue that performance is related to achieving the goals and satisfying the different constituents of an organization (hospital). Consequently organizational performance is a construct of multiple variables that are to be in balance.

Secondly, we realize that the performance is influenced by a lot of variables other than merely the design of the hospital. Therefore, we will focus on a more operational level on the performance of processes, on which level the influence of the design is most prominent and focus of the research is placed.

Organizational Performance: Construct of Multiple Variables to Be Balanced

Though developed in separate bodies of literature, the constructs of organizational effectiveness and performance seem to deal with the same issue of evaluating organizational practices. Some even propose to merge the two research areas [29, 30]. In describing the ultimate dependent variable in organization research [31], the construct of effectiveness has a much richer conceptual tradition from which we can learn a few basic ideas.

In organization theory the concept of effectiveness is given different meanings accompanied by different concepts of organization, different assumptions, operationalizations, methods, and techniques [32]. We adhere to the view that the different traditional effectiveness approaches are neither mutually exclusive nor antithetical [33]: the output-oriented *goal approach*, which focuses on how well the organization attains its goals [34]; the *system resource approach*, which focuses on [35] the ability of acquisition of scarce and valued resources [36]; and the *internal process approach* of effectiveness, which focuses on smooth internal functioning or organizational health [37, 38] and can be considered to be an approach for studying predictors of effectiveness [39].

We agree that ultimately the attainment of goals is the central factor in the study of (hospital) organizations [40], and as Perrow stated, goals are an important resource to an organization; they are a form of structure around which efforts are organized and thereby made relatively efficient, and clear goals help an organization employ its resources efficiently [41].

By continuing to ask how these goals are set, it is found that the goals *of* the organization are likely to emerge from the interaction of the goals, interests or expectations that the involved constituencies (or stakeholders) have *for* the organization [42]. This means that these goals are multivariable, sometimes even conflicting, and that trade-offs can be necessary.

More contemporary integrative approaches to effectiveness, such as the competing values (CV) approach [43] and the multiple constituency (MC) approach [44], recognize this and state that "different effectiveness statements can be made about the focal organization, reflecting the criterion sets of different individuals and groups" [44] (which are referred to as constituencies) and that "an organization is effective to the extent it satisfies the interests of one or more constituencies associated with the organization" [45].

Subsequently, effectiveness (or performance for that matter) should be used as an underlying construct for a model of what is denoted by effectiveness and that identifies the variables or measures taken into consideration [46]. It is constituted of variables from various organizational domains on which an organization must score in order to satisfy its constituencies or stakeholders.

In the area of strategic management, business performance or organizational performance is used to delineate a subset of the organizational effectiveness concept [47]. In this field, the dissatisfaction with traditional costing- and accounting-based and backward-looking performance measurement systems led to the development of performance measurement frameworks that are multidimensional and encourage a more balanced view [48]. Different authors proposed a balance between internal and external measures, financial and nonfinancial measures [49], measures of the results and their determinants [50], or between different perspectives in a balanced scorecard [51]. This balanced scorecard combines both financial as well as operational measures from the internal, customer, and innovation and learning perspective.

Though recent performance literature, just as effectiveness studies, reflects the multiple constituencies approach [52, 53] and the need for better understanding of performance is generally acknowledged, strategic studies with performance indicators based on stakeholders' evaluations are still hardly available [29, 30].

To summarize, we too adhere the belief that a combination of different measures is a fruitful way of demarcating performance and that only a balance between the different aspects leads to a satisfactory functioning or the "desired future state." In terms of guiding the process of design, what constitutes "performance" of a configuration or structure that is to be chosen is determined by the objectives or goals of an organization and includes variables from different domains, which in our view are a reflection of its stakeholders' interests. So, besides the contingencies of an organization, the involved stakeholders place their demands on the structuring of the organization and its processes. The notion of (hospital) stakeholder interests will be discussed more thoroughly in the next section.

Focus of the Construct on Performance of Processes

In our research into the design of hospitals we are searching for an operationalization of performance that can be used to evaluate building structures or design solutions. Central to our research, therefore, is how a desired performance, once determined, can be achieved, and how this can be done efficiently.

Therefore, we will refer to our adopted process-based view of organizations and focus on a more operational performance level that takes us beyond the black box approach and focuses on those key operational success factors [47] that lead to the performance and effectiveness of processes. Before relating the concept of performance more closely to hospital stakeholders, we will discuss our ideas about the performance of processes.

Øvretveit defined a three-dimensional approach to health service quality that also reflects the perspectives of primary constituents of a hospital [54, 55]:

- *Client quality*: whether clients (and carers) get what they want from a service;
- *Professional quality*: whether the service meets the patients' needs as defined by professional providers and referrers (outcome) and whether it correctly carries

out techniques and procedures that are believed to be necessary to meet patients' needs (process); and

• *Management quality*: the most efficient and productive use of resources within limits set by higher authorities.

In terms of these dimensions we have in mind the way the building structure can contribute to management quality as a requisite to achieve professional as well as client quality.

Adopting a process view of the organization like ours has some fundamental implications for organization performance measurement [56–58]. Clearly the choice of appropriate (performance) measures must be made in conjunction with the strategic goals of the firm and in close communication with a hospital's processes [59].

Running the risk of new terminology confusion, we want to stress that our performance of processes is not point for point the same as the process-based performance measures mentioned in a more general categorization of indicators of organizational effectiveness or quality, discerning those based on outcomes, those based on processes, and those based on structures [60, 61].

The performance of processes, as we argued, refers to the extent to which processes contribute to goal attainment and satisfaction of interests. A process performance measurement system would be characterized as a system that gathers—through a set of indicators—performance-relevant information on the business processes [62]. This means that linking the building structure to the performance of processes becomes something like linking structural characteristics or indicators to process measures, with outcome measures as strategic reference points.

A distinction between outcomes and predictors of outcomes, similar to the field of effectiveness studies, is also the basis for the Business Excellence Model, or European Foundation for Quality Management (EFQM) model [63]. Although the operationalization of the model can be criticized, the conceptual thought behind the model, in which nine categories of criteria are divided into *enablers* and *results* and the central idea is that a high-quality standard will be attained if attention is paid to these categories in a consistent manner, is a useful one.

Referring to the recent field of study of business process management [56] and the observation that quality improvement or performance measures are often linked to addressing the business in terms of "key business processes" [57, 64], a process-based performance reporting approach has been proposed using key performance indicators (KPI). Performance indicators should be aligned with processes before functions and should accomplish performance of entire processes instead of department or unit processes. While the outcomes (KPO) indicate or monitor the progress towards what is to be achieved in the key result areas identified in the organization's mission statement, the key performance drivers (KPD) are aligned with what happens "inside" business processes giving insight into what's influencing the outcomes [65, 66].

Some researchers in the Netherlands have tried to combine and categorize the performance indicators from different approaches into categories specifically aimed at hospitals. They found that a general framework can be generated but that it needs adjustments for each specific situation. They identified several categories: conditions for processes, technical quality of processes, relational quality in processes, information supporting processes, and production control or managing the logistics of processes [67].

Combining the approaches identified and referring to their terminology, we can state that in our view the structures of the building and accompanying organizational configuration are a crucial part of the capacity and conditions that determine the quality (relational, logistical) and performance (managerial) of processes and how well the hospital processes can drive the organization to achieving the desired outcomes (resulting in both professional and client quality).

The building structure shapes the hospital processes, which are essential for the organization to reach its objectives. The performance of processes is a measure of how well these contribute to the functioning of the organization and is constituted of indicators for different domains. The building structure should enable a balanced scorecard on the aspects constituting this performance of processes.

As implicitly recognized in naming aspects of relational quality or outcomes in terms of professional and client quality, and as argued before, these aspects must reflect the interests of the hospital constituents. So to design high-performance hospitals we will need to consider what constitutes this performance statement by relating to and recovering the interests of the parties directly involved, those who are meant to be the future users of the building. Our performance construct is therefore deduced from the set of interest of hospital stakeholders.

STAKEHOLDER INTERESTS: A BASIS FOR PERFORMANCE OF DESIGN

To determine a correct operationalization of our performance construct that will reflect the organizational goals, we will refer to the stakeholder theory. A very broadly accepted way of explaining the genesis of organizational goals is suggested by an examination of *stakeholder expectations*.

As mentioned earlier (in other words), each of an organization's stakeholders has somewhat different expectations for the organization that are related to the goals and interests of the various stakeholders themselves. The goals *of* the organization are likely to emerge from the interaction of these various goals *for* the organization [42].

To explain the concept of stakeholders, some of the relevant definitions and characterizations of stakeholders will be given, as used by different authors.

Short Introduction to the Concept of Stakeholders

Mitchell et al. [68] give an extensive overview of the various definitions of stakeholders that have been used in the literature. The definitions given by different authors differ in the emphasis put on certain aspects of the identification of stakeholders and their role or relationship towards the organization.

Stakeholders have been defined as broadly as "groups in relationship with an organization" [69], "groups to whom the corporation is responsible" [70], or those groups "on which the organization is dependent for its continued survival" [71]. The most commonly cited definition is given by Freeman, who defines a stakeholder as "any group or individual who can effect or is affected by the achievement of the organization's objectives" [72], which stresses the two possible directions of influence between an organization and its stakeholders. Though this distinction is a crucial one, it still leaves the definition and, therefore, the possible range of stakeholders very broad because theoretically every group or individual can affect or be affected by an organization. Narrower views define stakeholders in terms of their direct relevance to an organization's core economic interests [68]. In more instrumental views of the stakeholder concept the difference between "affecting" and affected groups is explicated and used to reduce the range of stakeholders taken into consideration to constituencies closely related to an organization.

A very useful addition to the stakeholder concept can be made from the multiple-constituency approach [44], by identifying stakeholders as the "constituencies that attempt to attain their goals by participating in a focal organization" [73, 74]. In this view the essence of participating is the exchange of contributions and inducements between stakeholders and the organization or between stakeholders through the focal organization [73, 75].

Stakeholders have a legitimate claim on the organization through their exchange relationship by supplying critical resources (contributions) and in return expecting their interests to be satisfied (by inducements) [74]. This reduces the group of stakeholders to directly involved parties that have power over the organization, which is dependent on them for their contributions—which are often scarce resources critical to the organization's survival [76]—and because of the fact that they can withhold their contribution. Such stakeholders can affect the achievement of goals of the organization and form the dominant coalition of that organization [77].

This approach corresponds with the distinction of internal and external stakeholders [78] and discerns primary from secondary stakeholders [79]. Primary, especially internal, stakeholders have a stake in a focal organization in which they participate to attain their own goals (and form the dominant coalition) and therefore have an interest in organizational survival. Stakeholders can then be identified based on the nature of the contributions or critical resources and the inducements, in a variety of forms satisfying the interests of stakeholders, that they exchange among themselves [75].

Hospital Performance by Stakeholders' Interests

We set out to use the concept of stakeholders as a means to determine what can be considered to be high performance in the case of hospitals. The concept of stakeholders has been used in different studies of hospitals. Savage et al. [80] noted that hospital executives in the United States must respond to an increasing number of active and powerful stakeholder groups. A study of hospital executives [81] identified the medical staffs, patients, hospital management, professional staffs, and boards of trustees as the five most important and powerful stakeholders for hospitals in the United States.

In response to government advocacy for greater attention to patient and other stakeholder requirements, suggestions for an integrated approach of stakeholder consultation were made in the United Kingdom. The all-encompassing approach should ensure that the perspectives of all key stakeholders are incorporated: the interests of the clients (patients), referrers (general practitioners), professionals (clinical staff, general practioners, health boards), and management (internally in hospitals and externally at the health board) [82]. Each of these stakeholder groups has its own expectations, and the hospital executives must set their performance goals to address the specific concerns of each group [80].

Freeman [72] and others argue that systematic managerial attention to stakeholder interests is crucial to a firm's success, and although empirical evidence about an association between orientation to (multiple) stakeholder interests and performance is not (yet) available, some form of association seems to be widely assumed in management literature [83]. Unlike the approach to investigating this relationship used by a lot of researchers who search for the effect of stakeholder management or orientation on performance, we have adopted in our research the approach that stakeholders and their interests, by definition, determine what constitutes performance.

In order to establish the performance aspects that ought to be taken

Figure 13.1
Different Categories of Hospital Stakeholders

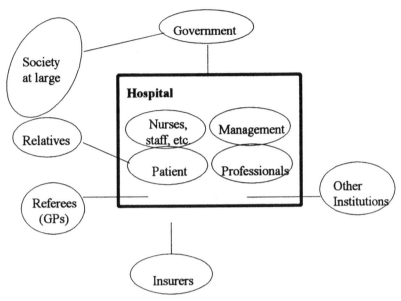

into consideration in a model of judging hospital design solutions, the interests of the stakeholders of a hospital organization are the natural starting point. A high-performance hospital will satisfy the interests of its most important, or primary, stakeholders.

A first overview of the stakeholders taken into consideration is shown in Figure 13.1.

Given that each stakeholder has its own unique set of expectations, needs, and values [84], a stakeholder map as proposed by Freeman (describing the wide range of stakeholder groups associated with companies) represents a wide and diverse range of interests [72], especially in the case of a hospital. Even using our narrower definition of primary stakeholders, and although there is considerable overlap and occasional compatibility in the expectations of the key stakeholders, they differ in terms of what concerns them most [85], and often their interests can be conflicting. In the preceding section we identified some categories of performance aspects that can be linked to the interests of different stakeholders from Figure 13.1.

Professionals will be interested in an environment in which they can do their work in a satisfying manner and achieve a high level of technical quality of outcomes. Management will be interested in efficient, logistically sound processes that reach a high level of managerial quality. In this chapter we will not discuss the different interests of all stakeholders in detail, but it may be obvious that a range of performance criteria can be generated by identifying these interests.

Normally, besides identifying stakeholders and their interests, the management of an organization has the difficult task of balancing the interest of the organization's stakeholders. This often means that certain trade-offs between incompatible goals have to be made. The claims that stakeholders can have on an organization are not all equally important, and management has to weigh the relative importance of these claims. The term "salience" is used for this. Salience is "the degree to which managers give priority to competing stakeholder claims" [68]. The way salience can be accounted for or the attributes that determine a stakeholder's salience is still a major subject of discussion [68, 75], but common to all concepts is the generally accepted fact that it is management's perception of these attributes that eventually determines a stakeholder's salience. In other words, it is a subjective measure. "Salience is in the eye of the beholder," so to speak. Therefore, it is not possible to give an a priori ranking to the importance of different stakeholder interests. More important, it is arbitrary to label the interests of one particular constituency a priori as the correct one because each represents a valid point of view in its own right [44].

The different sets of interests of the set of stakeholders are to be detected and combined and balanced in the overall set of performance aspects. Interaction of the stakeholders with the hospital executives results in performance goals that will partly overlap with the expectations of other stakeholders [86]. It is important to recognize that different groups of stakeholders may in fact be saying the same things in different ways, and it is crucial to be able to identify a set of priorities for strategic planning purposes [82].

This means that from an executive's perspective each performance goal must be designed to satisfy the concerns of multiple stakeholders [87]. This eventually must lead to a set of performance aspects that contains a "balanced scorecard" for hospital design in satisfying stakeholders' interests. In other words, the primary stakeholders have to recognize their interests in, and agree with, the multivariable operationalization of the concept of performance that will be used to determine the right design solution.

HOSPITAL DESIGN BY BALANCED STAKEHOLDER PERFORMANCE OF PROCESSES: A PROPOSAL

Hospital design has to facilitate diversity in the activities of the actors and cohesion within the different processes and units of organization to achieve a high level of compliance with the objectives of the hospital and its constituents. To help designers of hospitals find a configuration of

Figure 13.2
A Draft of Our "Balanced Scorecard" Approach for Careful Hospital Design

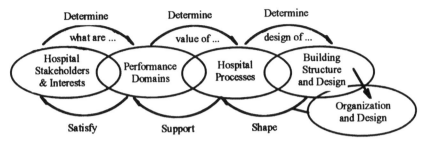

people, space, and technology that can meet the numerous requirements and demands, we propose a design approach that builds on articulated performance needs of various stakeholders on the level of processes. By doing so, we hope to explore the possibility of finding hospital designs that are consistent with the contingency propositions. At the same time, these designs must answer the demands that hospital stakeholders place on their structuring and processes. This will be done by creating a balanced scorecard of stakeholders' performance domains so that stakeholders will be satisfied by their participation in the various processes, which is crucial to functioning of the organization. This approach partly builds on research models proposed in operations management [28] and is depicted in Figure 13.2.

The starting point for design is therefore the identification of the varying interests of stakeholders in terms of performance domains. These are to be formulated on the level of processes and operationalized into the factors that lead to or drive performance. The stakeholders should approve of the representation of their combined interests in the set of performance indicators. This way these indicators of performance are the instrumental translation of the requirements that warrant a balance in the level of satisfaction of stakeholders' interests. These should then be used as the evaluation or judgmental criteria that guide the choices of design made to find the right combination of ordering principles for the configuration of the hospital.

To generate our framework of stakeholder interests and related performance domains, our research will involve different cases of hospitals developing new building plans. We will then operationalize this information into indicators of process performance that can be linked to the characteristics of the building structure.

The resulting framework will be tested for its usefulness. It has to offer new design teams assistance as an instrument for structural evaluation of design solutions. A proposed design can be judged on its consequences for the different performance domains by evaluation based on the indicators mentioned. In doing so it can assure that stakeholder interests have been consciously taken into consideration before deciding on a certain design. The balance of interests that is found will differ from case to case, depending on the relationships and influence of the stakeholders. But articulating these interests will help to create a consensus and make the choice a truly strategic one in the long term.

NOTES

[1] Sir Winston Churchill, in *The Times*, September 12, 1960.
[2] Burbidge, J. L., "Group Technology," in Wild, J. (Ed.), *International Handbook of Production and Operations Management* (London: Cassell Education Ltd., 1989).
[3] Muther, R., *Systematic Layout Planning* (Boston: Cahners, 1973).
[4] Van Buren, D. J., and Jan M. H. Vissers, "De kliniek en de polikliniek als produktielijnen, en clienten eerstelijnsvriendelijke ziekenhuisorganisatie," *Het ziekenhuis*, 17(3), 1987.
[5] Wulff, R. E., "Het ontwerpen van ziekenhuisorganisaties: Een onderzoek naar de organisatiestructuur van het algemene ziekenhuis" (Technical University of Eindhoven, 1996).
[6] Hammer, M., and J. Champy, *Reengineering the Corporation: A Manifesto for Business Revolution* (London: Nicholas Brealey, 1994).
[7] Ernst & Young & De ziekenhuisketen, "Eindrapportage project Verkorting van doorstroomtijden, herontwerp van zorgprocessen door BPR," Amersfoort, 2000.
[8] Suzaki, K., *The New Manufacturing Challenge* (New York: Free Press, 1987).
[9] Imai, M., *Kaizen, The Key to Japan's Competitive Success* (New York: Random House, 1986).
[10] Scarparo, S., "Clinical Governance: An Instrument for Bringing Quality and Efficiency Together?" paper presented at the 1st HCTM Hospital of the Future conference proceedings, Enschede, The Netherlands, 2001.
[11] Ruffini, F.A.J., *Production System Design: From Practice to Theory* (Enschede, the Netherlands: University of Twente, 1999).
[12] Donaldson, L., *In Defence of Organizational Theory: A Reply to the Critics* (Cambridge: Cambridge University Press, 1985).
[13] Lawrence, P. R., J. W. Lorsch, and J. S. Garrison, *Organization and Environment: Managing Differentiation and Integration* (Boston: Harvard Business School Press, 1967).
[14] Hattinga Verschure, J.C.M., *Patient Ziekenhuis Gezondheidszorg op weg naar 2000* (Amsterdam/Brussels: Agon Elsevier, 1971).
[15] Van Buren, D. J., and J.M.H. Vissers, "De kliniek en de polikliniek als produktielijnen, en client- en eerstelijnsvriendelijke ziekenhuisorganisatie," in Hoorn, J. W., J. Lettink, H. Van Tuijl, J.M.H. Vissers, and G. De Vries (Eds.), *Structurering en beheersing van zorgprocessen, Bedrijfskundig instrumentarium voor de ziekenhuismanager* (Lochem: De Tijdstroom, 1991).
[16] Kalay, Yehuda E., "Performance-Based Design," *Automation in Construction*, 8(4), 1999, 395–409.

[17] Lettink, J., "Ziekenhuisorganisatie en managementinstrumenten in historisch perspectief," in Hoorn, J. W., J. Lettink, H. Van Tuijl, J.M.H. Vissers, and G. De Vries (Eds.), *Structurering en beheersing van zorgprocessen: Bedrijfskundig instrumentarium voor de ziekenhuismanager* (Lochem: De Tijdstroom, 1991).

[18] Mintzberg, H., *The Structuring of Organizations: A Synthesis of the Research* (Englewood Cliffs, NJ: Prentice-Hall, 1979).

[19] Woodward, J., *Industrial Organization: Theory and Practice* (London: Oxford University Press, 1965).

[20] Khandwalla, Prahid N., "Viable and Effective Organizational Designs of Firms," *Academy of Management Journal*, 19, 1973, 481–495.

[21] Jansen, H.F.A., C.P.C. Bremen ter Stege, and F. Doeleman, "Samenhang van de zorgverlening. Afstemming binnen primaire proces van de gezondheidszorg," *M en O* 5, 1985, 36–49.

[22] Jansen, P.G.W., "Op weg naar een empirische bedrijfskunde," *Bedrijfskunde*, 66(1), 1994, 45–50.

[23] Doty, H. D., W. Glick, and G. P. Huber, "Fit, Equifinality and Organizational Effectiveness: A Test of Two Configurational Theories," *Academy of Management Journal*, 36(6), 1993, 1196–1250.

[24] Gresov, Christopher, and Robert Drazin, "Equifinality: Functional Equivalence in Organization Design," *Academy of Management Review*, 22(2), 1997, 403–428.

[25] Draaijer, D. J., *Market-Oriented Manufacturing Systems: Theory and Practice* (Twente, The Netherlands: Universiteit Twente, 1993).

[26] Draaijer, Domien J., and Harry Boer, "Designing Market-Oriented Production Sytems: Theory and Practice," *Integrated Manufacturing Systems*, 6(4), 1995, 4–15.

[27] Child, John, "Organizational Structure, Environment and Performance: The Role of Strategic Choice," *Sociology*, 6, 1972, 1–22.

[28] Ruffini, Frans A. J., Harry Boer, and Maarten J. Van Riemsdijk, "Organisation Design in Operations Management," *International Journal of Operations and Production Management*, 20(7), 2000, 860–879.

[29] Glunk, U., and C.P.M. Wilderom, *Organizational Effectiveness = Corporate Performance? Why and How Two Research Traditions Need to Be Merged* (Tilburg, The Netherlands: Tilburg University, 1996).

[30] Glunk, U., and C.P.M. Wilderom, *High Performance on Multiple Domains: Operationalizing the Stakeholder Approach to Evaluate Organizations* (Tilburg, The Netherlands: Tilburg University, 1998).

[31] Cameron, K. S., and D. A. Whetten, *Organizational Effectiveness: A Comparison of Multiple Models* (San Diego: Academic Press, 1983).

[32] Cameron, Kim S., "Measuring Organizational Effectiveness in Institutes of Higher Education," *Administrative Science Quarterly*, 23, 1978, 604–632.

[33] Weimer, J., and M.J. Van Riemsdijk, *A New Magical Lamp to Rub? The Multiple Constituency Approach: A Potential Useful Framework for Research on the Organizational Effectiveness Construct* (Enschede, The Netherlands: University of Twente, 1997).

[34] Price, J. L., "The Study of Organizational Effectiveness," *The Sociological Quarterly*, 13, 1972, 3–15.

[35] Cunningham, J., "A System-Resource Approach for Evaluating Organizational Effectiveness," *Human Relations*, 31, 1978, 631–656.

[36] Yuchtman, E., and S. E. Seashore, "A System Resource Approach to Organizational Effectiveness," *American Sociological Review*, 32, 1967, 891–903.

[37] Bennis, W. G., "The Concept of Organizational Health," Bennis, W. G. (Ed.), *Changing Organizations* (New York: McGraw-Hill, 1966).

[38] Daft, R. L., *Organization Theory and Design* (St. Paul, MN: West Publishing, 1992).

[39] Bluedorn, A. C., "Cutting the Gordian Knot: A Critique of the Effectiveness Tradition in Organizational Research," *Sociology and Social Research*, 64, 1980, 477–496.

[40] Gross, E., "The Definition of Organizational Goals," *British Journal of Sociology*, 20, 1969, 277–294.

[41] Perrow, C., *Organizational Analysis: A Sociological View* (Belmont, CA: Wadsworth, 1970).

[42] Ullrich, R. A., and G. F. Wieland, *Organization Theory and Design* (Homewood, IL: Richard D. Irwin, 1980).

[43] Quinn, R. E., and J. Rohrbaugh, "A Spatial Model of Effectiveness Criteria: Towards a Competing Values Approach to Organizational Analysis," *Management Science*, 29, 1983, 363–377.

[44] Conolly, T., E. J. Conlon, and S. J. Deutsch, "Organizational Effectiveness: A Multiple-Constituency Approach," *Academy of Management Review*, 2, 1980, 211–217.

[45] Tsui, Anne S., "A Multiple-Constituency Model of Effectiveness: An Empirical Examination at the Human Resource Subunit Level," *Administrative Science Quarterly*, 35, 1990, 458–483.

[46] Campbell, J. P., "On the Nature of Organizational Effectiveness," in Goodman, P. S., and J. M. Pennings (Eds.), *New Perspectives on Organizational Effectiveness* (San Francisco: Jossey-Bass, 1977), pp. 13–55.

[47] Venkatraman, N., and Vasudevan Ramanujam, "Measurement of Business Performance in Strategy Research: A Comparison of Approaches," *Academy of Management Review*, 11(4), 1986, 801–814.

[48] Bourne, Mike C. S., John F. Mills, Mark Wilcox, Andy D. Neely, and Ken W. Platts, "Designing, Implementing and Updating Performance Measurement Systems," *International Journal of Operations and Production Management*, 20(7), 2000, 754–771.

[49] Keegan, D. P., R. G. Eiler, and C. R. Jones, "Are Your Performance Measures Obsolete?" *Management Accounting*, 12, 1989, 45–50.

[50] Fitzgerald, L., R. Johnston, T. J. Brignall, R. Silvestro, and C. Voss, *Performance Measurement in Service Business* (London: The Chartered Institute of Management Accountants, 1991).

[51] Kaplan, Robert S., and David P. Norton, "The Balanced Scorecard—Measures That Drive Performance," *Harvard Business Review*, 70, 1992, 71–79.

[52] Chakravarthy, Balaji S., "Measuring Strategic Performance," *Strategic Management Journal*, 7, 1986, 437–458.

[53] Doyle, P., "Setting Business Objectives and Measuring Performance," *Journal of General Management*, 20(2), 1994, 1–19.

[54] Øvretveit, J., *Health Service Quality* (Oxford: Blackwell Scientific Press, 1992).

[55] Øvretveit, John, "Total Quality Management in European Healthcare," *International Journal of Health Care Quality Assurance*, 13(2), 2000, 74–79.

[56] Harrington, H. J., *Business Process Improvement: The Breakthrough Strategy for Total Quality, Productivity, and Competitiveness* (New York: McGraw-Hill, 1991).

[57] Jones, C. R., "Improving Your Key Business Processes," *Total Quality Management*, 6, 1994, 25–29.

[58] Walsh, Paul, "Managing Performance Indicators: Part II. What Process Was That?" *Benchmark*, 11, 1995, 26–27.

[59] Kaplan, Robert S., and David P. Norton, "The Balanced Scorecard—Measures That Drive Performance," *Harvard Business Review*, 70, 1992, 71–79.

[60] Donabedian, A., "Evaluating the Quality of Medical Care," *Milbank Memorial Fund Quarterly*, 44(194), 1966, 196–214.

[61] Scott, W. R., "Effectiveness of Organizational Effectiveness Studies," in Goodman, P. S., and J. M. Pennings (Eds.), *New Perspectives on Organizational Effectiveness* (San Francisco: Jossey-Bass, 1977).

[62] Kueng, Peter, "Process Performance Measurement System: A Tool to Support Process-Based Organizations," *Total Quality Management*, 11(1), 2000, 67–85.

[63] European Foundation for Quality Management (EFQM), *Total Quality Management: The European Model for Self-Appraisal* (Eindhoven, The Netherlands: EFQM, 1992).

[64] Peters, J., "Operationalizing Total Quality: A Business Approach," *Total Quality Management*, 6(4), 1994, 29–33.

[65] Walsh, Paul K., "Finding Key Performance Drivers: Some New Tools," *Total Quality Management*, 7(5), 1996, 509–519.

[66] Neely, Andy D., John F. Mills, Ken W. Platts, A. Hugh Richards, Mike J. Gregory, Mike C. S. Bourne, and Mike Kennerly, "Performance Measurement System Design: Developing and Testing a Process-Based Approach," *International Journal of Operations and Production Management*, 20(10), 2000, 1119–1145.

[67] Van der Bij, J., and Jan M. H. Vissers, "Monitoring Health-Care Processes: A Framework for Performance Indicators," *International Journal of Health Care Quality Assurance*, 12(5), 1999, 214–221.

[68] Mitchell, R. K., B. R. Agle, and D. J. Wood, "Toward a Theory of Stakeholder Identification and Salience: Defining the Principle of Who and What Really Counts," *Academy of Management Review*, 22, 1997, 853–886.

[69] Thompson, J. K., S. L. Wartick, and H. L. Smith, "Integrating Corporate Social Responsibility and Stakeholder Management: Implications for a Research Agenda in Small Business," *Research in Corporate Social Performance and Policy*, 12, 1991, 207–230.

[70] Alkhafaji, A. F., *A Stakeholder Approach to Corporate Governance: Managing in a Dynamic Environment* (Westport, CT: Quorum Books, 1989).

[71] Stanford Research Institute, cited in Freeman, R. E., *Strategic Management: A Stakeholder Approach* (Boston: Pitman, 1984).

[72] Freeman, R. E., *Strategic Management: A Stakeholder Approach* (Boston: Pitman, 1984).

[73] March, J. G., and H. A. Simon, *Organizations* (New York: John Wiley & Sons, 1958).

[74] Hill, Charles W. L., and Gareth R. Jones, "Stakeholder-Agency Theory," *Journal of Management Studies*, 29(2), 1992, 131–154.

[75] Weimer, J., and M. J. Van Riemsdijk, *What's at Stake? A Step Closer Toward a Theory of Stakeholder Identification and Salience* (Enschede, The Netherlands: University of Twente, 1998).

[76] Pfeffer, J., and G. L. Salancik, *The External Control of Organizations* (New York: Harper & Row, 1978).

[77] Thompson, J. D., *Organizations in Action: Social Science Bases of Administrative Theory* (New York: McGraw-Hill, 1967).

[78] Mitroff, I. I., *Stakeholders of the Organizational Mind* (San Francisco: Jossey-Bass, 1983).

[79] Clarkson, M.B.E., "A Stakeholder Framework for Analyzing and Evaluating Corporate Social Performance," *Academy of Management Review*, 20, 1995, 92–117.

[80] Savage, Grant T., John D. Blair, and M. Benson, "Urban-Rural Hospital Affiliations: Assessing Control, Fit, and Stakeholder Issues Strategically," *Health Care Management Review*, 17(1), Winter 1992, 35–49.

[81] Fottler, Myron D., John D. Blair, Carlton J. Whitehead, M. D. Laus, and Grant T. Savage, "Who Matters to Hospitals and Why? Assessing Key Stakeholders," *Hospital and Health Services Administration*, 34(4), Winter 1989, 525–546.

[82] Curry, Adrienne, Sandra Stark, and Lesley Summerhill, "Patient and Stakeholder Consultation in Healthcare," *Managing Service Quality*, 9(5), 1999, 327–336.

[83] Donaldson, T., and L. E. Preston, "The Stakeholder Theory of the Corporation: Concepts, Evidence, and Implications," *Academy of Management Review*, 20, 1995, 65–91.

[84] King, W. R., and D. I. Cleland, *Strategic Planning* (New York: Van Nostrand Reinhold, 1979).

[85] Fottler, Myron D., "Health Care Organizational Performance: Present and Future Research," *Journal of Management*, 13(2), 1987, 179–203.

[86] Blair, John D., Grant T. Savage, and Carlton J. Whitehead, "A Strategic Approach for Negotiating with Hospital Stakeholders," *Health Care Management Review*, 14, 1989, 13–23.

[87] Counte, Michael A., "Improving Hospital Performance: Issues in Assessing the Impact of TQM Activities," *Hospital and Health Services Administration*, 40(1), 1995, 80–94.

Chapter 14

Linkage of User (Tenant) Demands to the (Physical) Building Facility

Tomas Engström, Lars Göran Bergqvist,
and Jan-Erik Gasslander

INTRODUCTION

This chapter recapitulates selected experiences and methods emanating from the design of a number of assembly systems and gives a brief outline of some general principles existing within the automotive industry regarding the organization of extensive industrial projects. These experiences and methods are embedded in the author's professional work as a senior researcher, working in close cooperation with practitioners in the Swedish automotive industry during the last 25 years.

From this platform, the authors argue and illustrate how to link the (physical) building facility to demands generated by the activities contained within the (physical) building facility. This is achieved by illuminating the linkage of the (physical) building facility to user (tenant) demands through a recommended building design (and construction) process, using a comparison of the healthcare sector characteristics versus the automotive industry's and the university's characteristics.

To design building facilities in congruence with user (tenant) demands and to support activities contained in the building has, in fact, proved to be intriguing, according to the three authors' recent mutual experiences. This experience concerns design of building facilities within the university. The authors suggest that a building design process in accordance with the principles and praxis used within the automotive industry will result in a recommended building design process that is continuously monitored at a number of checkpoints ("gates") defined beforehand. This chapter also briefly describes some constructive measures to be used for linking user (tenant) demands to the (physical) building facility. The authors also describe some practical means for design of public building facilities, including healthcare building facilities.

To conclude, applying principles and praxis from industrial product development processes and assembly system design to the building design process implies the need to shift focus from the physical building (i.e., transforming the building functions into a more abstract artifact).

This calls for a more far-reaching product specification of the (physical) building facility, stretching from the beginning of the building design process to the user (tenant) and corresponding to automotive product specification in the form of product data included in a product structure. This so-called virtual artifact (product specification based on appropriate product data), which is changing continuously, undergoes reform in relation to a shifting environment and user (tenant) demands.

Not until the input for reformation is monitored and organized in quite a different way from the common praxis in the building trade today will it be possible to create appropriate public building facilities. This will then form one vital ingredient of the "hospital of the future."

THE AUTOMOTIVE EXPERIENCE

University and healthcare buildings are, in most cases, examples of public building facilities. As a result, their construction is usually controlled by various governmental regulations and is also closely coupled to a political context.

Two authors' experiences (25 years) in the Swedish automotive industry concerning principles and praxis from industrial product development processes and assembly system design have recently been contrasted to the logic of the building trade through experiences common to all three authors regarding three cases of design (and construction) of public buildings within the Swedish university [1]. These experiences are briefly reported below. The third author has experience (20 years) in the design of various public buildings in Sweden, including healthcare buildings. The authors' joint university experience has been reported in [2] and [3].

In this chapter, the merits of an overarching comparison between branches/trades are underlined. This is especially vital concerning various aspects of the building trade, which in Sweden has been criticized for producing far too expensive, low-quality building facilities, not fully suited for the user (tenant) (see recent criticism [4]).

Using the automotive industry and the university as representative extremes, this chapter will discuss the design of building facilities, that is, hinting at how to organize the building design process in order to establish a linkage of user (tenant) demands to the (physical) building facility. The result will provide insights applicable to the healthcare sector.

Example 1

The photographs in Figure 14.1, from the Volvo Uddevalla plant design, show the components in a decomposed Volvo 740-model. Each photograph corresponds to one-eighth of an automobile, approximately one hour's assembly work. By positioning the removed components beside each other according to position within the automobile body, they helped illuminate the assembly work in a plant where one-eighth of an automobile was assembled in eight separate assembly workshops in series as is schematically shown below in Figure 14.1. The suggested assembly system design comprised workstation systems with three operators resulting in 20 minutes' cycle time, a division of labor suggested by the manufacturing engineers at Volvo, since it was assumed to be the maximum economically viable cycle time. This made it evident that such a plant would require either large intermediate buffers between each assembly workshop or a constant shifting of operators according to time differences between individual products and product variants; consider, for example, the components needed for an air conditioner added to the components shown in the photographs. This way the suggested division of labor would imply extra space requirements and system losses as well as a degradation of the product perception by basing it on only one-eighth of an automobile.

These photographs proved to be valuable when formulating and communicating one of the author's specific work structuring principles and methods. The removed components were, for example, organized according to detailed product data included in a product structure. In the case of the automotive industry, it was a matter of utilizing existing product data from the traditional design-oriented product structure complemented by a newly developed assembly-oriented product structure. The latter product structure is a hierarchical product structure describing the vehicle from an assembly point of view, thus forming a new product specification necessary for radical reformation of the traditional assembly line [5].

These specific work structuring principles and methods were used both for the design of several assembly systems as well as for running and maintaining the product data during the full-scale manufacturing, thus forming an unavoidable platform for revision of the product during the operation's (e.g., a plant) total life. In all respects this meant exceeding the building design process time perspective, including giving quite another meaning to design and product specification, irrespective of whether it is a matter of manufacturing of vehicles or design of buildings.

It also ought to be noted that specific labels were fixed to each component representing various product variants and complemented by small paper cards guiding the disassembly. These cards were positioned on the tables next to the removed components and comprised an illustration of the assembly work, and the appropriate product variant codification, and so forth. Thus it was possible to shift between the physical products' components and the product data in order to create a new description of the work being performed within the building. In the Volvo Uddevalla case, like in other of the authors' cases referred to, it was a matter of long-term engagement for the researchers during a long period of time (four to five years).

Figure 14.1
Components in a Decomposed Volvo 740-Model

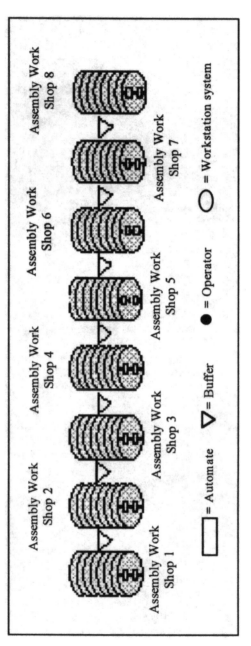

On top there is a disassembled automobile where the components are positioned on the floor according to their position in the automobile body as an example of one specific method for creating a more appropriate product specification, in the form of product data included in a product structure. This formed the base for a radical reformation of the traditional assembly line. At the bottom there is an assembly system design schematized where one-eighth of an automobile is assembled in parallel workstation systems holding two automobiles and three operators assembling the components shown above. This practical measure was a practical way of linking the planned activities to the (physical) building facility.

THE THREE AUTHORS' RECENT EXPERIENCES WITH DESIGN OF UNIVERSITY BUILDINGS

According to the authors' experiences concerning the design of university buildings, the importance of user (tenant) participation in the building design process, comprising the process, program, planning, building, and maintenance phases in accordance with Figure 14.3 (seen later in this chapter), must be underlined and carried by means of formalized methods (e.g., [6, 7]). Such formalized methods were to some extent used earlier for public buildings during the period when there was an overall responsible governmental authority in Sweden (i.e., The Swedish National Board of Public Building, Kungliga Byggnadsstyrelsen, [8]).

The critical function of a correctly designed and utilized building program, as an integrated part of the more traditional building design documentation, must be emphasized. This program must be constructed and communicated in the early phases of the building design process and ought to be accepted by all persons involved. Such a building program constitutes the platform for the later phases of the building design process. It must also be stressed that the building program ought to include all costs, even those costs that are not directly related to the building in the early estimations included in the planning phase. This might, for example, comprise costs such as rent for temporary premises for the user (tenant) who has to move around on the campus and the cost of lost earnings due to discrepancies in the provision of premises.

The ways of providing premises within the university are definitely questionable. The recent mutual experiences from the authors relate to three cases. In each case user (tenant) demands have been neglected and, in some cases, the user (tenant) has been forced to finance his/her own engineering and architecture expert advice in order to have some influence on the buildings projected, all in conflict with the university property manager. This might seem like a severe statement, but according to the authors' professional work, which has involved several large industrial projects embracing the building design process, the adduced design of university buildings deserves such criticism.

All these anomalies emanate from the property owner (i.e., the university), whose qualifications as a customer of building facilities have proved to be low. Nevertheless, the resulting costs for renting the premises are perplexing [9]. Consequently, the extreme rent, exceeding 2,700 Swedish Krones per square meter year for premises that are by no means suited for the user (tenant), is definitely outrageous.

Note that comparable premises rented outside the university would cost a quarter to a half of this price. One reason for this is the property manager's (a separate organization from the university) striving for a

Figure 14.2
Layout of the New Premises at Chalmers University of Technology, School of Technology Management and Economics

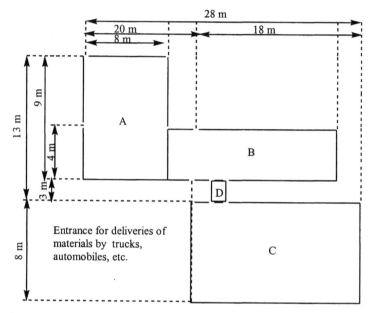

A = Offices of various sizes from one to three persons.

B = Combined office and laboratory (i.e., space possible for light mechanical and electrical work).

C = Laboratory for heavy mechanical work but also possible to use as an office.

D = Glassed crossing between the buildings containing offices and the building harboring laboratories. This was necessary since old buildings were utilized and the vibrations from the metal cutting machines are not allowed to affect the work in the other building.

universal building that can be rented to anyone in the future—a desire that resulted in the rejection of a design for low-cost, less specified premises. This preposterousness has to some extent been circumvented by other means as is exemplified in Figure 14.2. For a more detailed description of these three cases of the idiosyncrasies of building design processes within the university, see [3].

Example 2

This example examines the layout of the new premises at Chalmers University of Technology, School of Technology Management and Economics; in this case the office and experimental laboratory for Materials Handling Research Group at the Department of Transportation and Logistics. These premises have an internal flexibility that is gained through (1) the combined office and laboratory, which could be utilized either as office space, as a laboratory, or as a combination of the two; (2) possibilities to cut off at various positions along the line from A to C and to create offices from both ends; and (3) the use of various sizes of office rooms, in one case a room less than 10 square meters, for temporary work and guests, which also improves flexibility. Note, however, that this has by no means been a smooth building design process. Some severe restrictions still exist. For example, the building permit does not allow regular transports to the experimental laboratory. This layout was, on the initiative of the authors, designed to gain internal flexibility that ought to be considered in other cases. From the early phases, however, this flexibility was by no means defined in the building program and thus did not affect the total building design process except for this specific premise.

NOTED DISCREPANCIES AND CONSTRUCTIVE MEASURES

During the adduced design of university buildings the authors have had the following experiences worth noting:

1. The existence of time pressure, including intermittent straining of the user resources, which is sometimes utilized by building design representatives who have access to all the detailed information concerning the premises, long-term experiences from similar building projects, and a general survey of the specific building project. This advantage is not present for the users (tenants), who are provided with incomplete information and forced to decide under time pressure without realizing the consequences of the decisions on their future operation.

2. The occurrence of unclear responsibilities between building design representatives and property owner (i.e., the university represented by their own Division for Estates and Facilities Management) where some specific decision makers (i.e., university board and the headmaster) function as customers of building facilities. It is important that the involved responsible personnel and their respective roles are defined in detail beforehand. The building design processes have encountered various critical situations in two of the cases. It has, for example, been unclear what the written commitments required from the user (tenant) mean and how many such commitments a user (tenant) is supposed to meet. The building project representatives have also neglected to inform the user (tenant) who the actual receiver is and have covered up what the consequences would be if the completed (physical) building facility did not fulfill the users' (tenant) requirements. The latter aspect is an absolute necessity to enlighten the responsible persons within the university. This has not been the case during the experiences referred to here. In most cases the appropriate persons from the users' side have not been involved in the participation process, since the responsible persons for research and education activities usually are occupied. In addition, no slack or designated resources for participating were included in the building design

processes referred to (i.e., in the early cost estimates, included in the planning phase, no such resources were considered).

3. The stiff-legged formalism in the formulation of building functions derived from building design representatives regarding routines and practices, including vague and overarching directives from the property owner (i.e., the university), functioning as a customer of building facilities represented by their own Division for Estates and Facilities Management, which works on the directives of the university board and the headmaster. This is why, as mentioned above, lower quality premises have not been considered in the cases referred to. There has been an explicit policy that all rooms should have the same high standard, independent of use.

Another peculiarity was the building design representatives' refusal to utilize any form of schematization of material flow [10], the lack of specified criteria for exploitation due to communality between various departments, as well as not caring the least about aspects like size of entrances, door heights, loads on floor, and so forth. Only through the initiatives of the users were these vital aspects included in the building design process, in some cases at a phase that was far too late. The resulting costs for renting the projected premises are perplexing. Thus it is strange that the formal mechanism for distributing these costs among the users has not been debated or clarified.

These facts led to insecurity. Even though for a long time it has been acknowledged that the extreme rent would not be covered by the 10 percent added to the externally financed research projects, the consequences thereof are still not defined. In the near future this might lead to departments within the university needing laboratories, for instance, and having to close down their activities because of this need. Alternatively, disciplines requiring substantially smaller premises will be forced to finance activities in need of laboratories, and so forth. Another restriction worth noting concerning Swedish governmental research foundations is that they do not accept increased administrative costs. Thereby the researchers have to conceal these costs in the calculation when applying for research grants in various ways.

4. The fact that user (tenant) participation and dialogue are carried through by means of insufficient methods based on inadequate information, which means that, for example, the architects have neglected to clarify, or been hindered in clarifying, fundamental aspects of user (tenant) demands. The architects have produced assumed layouts without practical relevance and thereby failed to recognize different users' (tenants') varying demands. Elementary demands like the need to bring materials into laboratories and workshops and various aspects of security (e.g., the choice of doors, door frames, and windows) have not been recognized. The traditional building documentation, however, calls for

expertise to be examined. This would be observed if user (tenant) participation is called for.

In all the cases referred to, most of the users (tenants) lacked sufficient insights in what data, according to the building trade praxis and routines, they ought to request for their participation and for formulating appropriate written commitments. Binders, for example, comprising building permit, building program, cost calculations, and organization charts clarifying responsibilities of the building design representatives, were lacking and never asked for by the users (tenants). They did not, by the way, have sufficient experience to understand and survey all the phases of the building design process in accordance with Figure 14.3.

5. The lack of routines for feedback to the user (tenant) concerning how and which building function was insufficient or lacking totally; in none of the adduced cases did such an appropriate mechanism exist to continuously secure user (tenant) demands. In one of the three cases such a mechanism was constructed by users' (tenant) initiatives, as is explained below, and eventually led to somewhat acceptable premises after a long period of complications and extensive extraordinary engagement.

The experiences described above are, according to the authors' experiences, possible to attend to by constructive measures. Otherwise, expensive and costly actions, after the building is completed, will be necessary under time pressure, possibly also resulting in legal matters regarding, for example, whom to blame and whom to charge with the additional costs.

Fortunately, the building design representatives usually carry out the actions required if their extra costs are paid, which generally are extremely high in the late phases of a building project. Naturally, the users (tenants) will in most cases not be willing to finance demands agreed upon during the planning phase and delays due to insufficient design.

Nevertheless, if this is the case, the building design documentation will be very important. It also ought to be noted that the state of the art reported above is in accordance with the observation made by, for example, Statens Arbetsmiljönämnd [11] 20 years ago.

The authors have, with some success, used some constructive measures during one of the cases referred to here. In the other cases some of the authors were consulted during the planning phase leading to the utilization of some of the measures recommended, while others were neglected by the building design representatives in spite of sharply formulated written commitments.

The constructive measures recommended, and used by the authors, were:

1. The help of professional external support for users (tenants), for example, experts within the building trade but operating freely outside the purview of the building project's representatives engaged by the uni-

versity. In one of the cases a consultant (university-trained engineer and architect) assisted during a two-year period, functioning as a contact between the users (tenants) and the building design representatives; the users (tenants) solely financed him. Due to various reasons it became evident early in the building design process that it was important for the users (tenants) to analyze their demands and to have consequences judged or illuminated by various experts. This proved to be the only way to transform user (tenant) demands into building functions.

2. The use of a number of standardized room function programs (specification of building functions comprised in various rooms). In these room function programs the deviations from a stipulated standard were registered. In none of the three cases referred to were any such programs provided by the building design representatives.

3. The need for developing a number of illustrative examples and checklists intended for both users (tenants) and the building design representatives as well as for the top managers within the university who were not familiar with the logic and details of a building project. In one of the cases, for example, it was necessary for the user to utilize a popular science article describing aspects on electrical security [12] in order to illustrate critical knowledge for the building project representatives which, in fact, ought to be available within a technical university. This topic was debated 18 months before this article posed the problem and gave appropriate references.

4. The necessity to construct a form aimed at the building project representatives for their own self-control. According to Swedish law, a formal statement by the official safety representative for a place of work is required before a building can be occupied. One of the authors was, in fact, the official safety representative. Thus it was possible to elaborate an appropriate form that functioned as an official dialogue instrument (i.e., a written statement as a formal self-account from the building design representatives). Thereby various vital anomalies were brought forward, forming the ingredients for later resolution of specific problem areas by independent expertise. This form comprised, for example, questions like: Do the building facilities fulfill the adoption requirements for disabled people according to specified laws? Do the building facilities fulfill the legislation regarding recycling of material used in accordance with specified laws? Are there any remaining discrepancies affecting user (tenant)–planned activities connected to the building facilities? The choice of answers was "yes," "no," and "don't know."

5. On-site inspections by the user (tenant). The inspecting users were supported by their own experts during selected moments of the building design process, the fulfillment of user (tenant) demands were controlled. The results from the inspections were entered in minutes. Concerning selected aspects, it proved necessary for the user (tenant) to contact the

local building board and other experts to clarify specific topics and regulations. These clarifications concerned various aspects on which the building design representatives earlier had been vague even though the topics had repeatedly been brought forward. One example is that the sewer of the laboratories called for measures to separate oil from water. The ethics of and the information from the building design representatives proved to be questionable—for example, making false statements that easily could be checked by the user (tenant) during various meetings, something that occasionally occurred, did not create confidence.

6. The consideration of safety aspects, which in one of the adduced cases proved necessary to handle in a practical way. After the users (tenant) had moved into the premises, it proved necessary to arrange destructive tests. This activity, comprising six selected objects, was supervised by representatives from the property owner, users (tenant), safety experts from the university, and work environment representatives. These tests showed that some of the safety aspects were indisputably inferior. In fact, the destructive tests proved that it was possible to gain access to the premises in six selected trials in between 20 seconds and 5 minutes without setting of the alarm installed. According to agreement with the insurance company, the ability to resist break-ins with conventional hand tools for a minimum of 10 minutes is required to make the premises sufficiently safe.

This unsatisfying degree of safety was evident even though earlier, during the six months when the premises were used, the building design representatives had asserted that this was not the case. No verification mechanism for attainment of the defined safety level determined in the building design was considered. The destructive tests were initiated at one of the authors' (tenant) initiatives. These destructive tests resulted in a written statement defining the object, tools required and time required, combined with video recordings, of which the latter were utilized for dialogues with selected entrepreneurs, responsible for doors and door frames, glass partitions, locks and locking devices, and so forth. The result was that several doors and doorframes had to be replaced and that some glass partitions had to be modified (turned around, since they were fitted with the screwed rails facing public areas) or substituted.

Some of the authors had tried, but not succeeded, to investigate the blurred relationships between user (tenant) and building design representatives. In one of the cases referred to, it was a requisite for the user (tenant) to hire external building experts and pay for them, thus getting help from a retired top manager, earlier responsible for building facilities in a large international Swedish company. The only regret was not having done this much earlier. The building design process, however, had been going on for one and a half years before this remedy was employed as the only obvious way to at least get somewhat acceptable premises.

SOME ASPECTS OF A RECOMMENDED BUILDING DESIGN PROCESS

It might be argued that some frames of references from the automotive industry have already been transferred to the building trade. For example, the term facility management has recently been coined as an umbrella term for various initiatives. However, even though some selected terms from industry may cross over, the profound concept and principles have not yet been recognized within the building trade.

Even though, according to IVA [13], terms like product development, which has a specific meaning within the automotive industry, are now used in building design, this does not mean that user (tenant) demands are fully recognized in practice. It might also be noted that the need for further use of industrial frames of references is brought forward by the Swedish Union [14], which underlines that the term "value chains" is used within industry at large, but not in the building trade.

Briefly explained, the industrial product development process implies that the assumed product functions are defined, specified, and thereafter split up between designers before the physical product is used by the final customer (i.e., the owner of the vehicle). Intersected between these activities, a number of "loops" occur, which comprise both digital and physical mock-ups and prototypes used for verifying the linkage between user (tenant) demands and the complete product on the market.

Even after marketing (when the product is owned by the final customer), the product specification in the form of product data included in a product structure is cherished. This product structure forms a platform for implementing the product (design change orders) and introducing new product variants—as well as for exploiting carryover components, "securing" various legal aspects of the product (in the case of vehicles in the form of safety and emission standards), and so forth. These procedures are in contrast to the building design process in which the building design representatives leave a specific building design in order to repeat the procedure elsewhere, thus leaving the user (tenant) and the property owner alone in the completed building facility.

Figure 14.3 comprises the process, program, planning, building, and maintenance phases. It must, as is the case in extensive projects within the automotive industry, be continuously checked by a number of checkpoints ("gates") defined beforehand. No further work within the building design ought to proceed until the agreed criteria at the checkpoints are fulfilled [15].

This comparison implies the need for a more far-reaching product

Figure 14.3
The Building Design Process

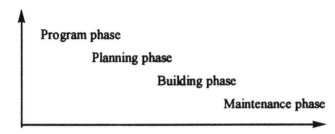

The phases in a building design process according to the three authors' experiences.

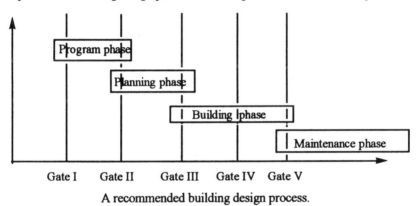

A recommended building design process.

specification of building facilities, stretching from the beginning of the building design process to the user (tenant). However, there are some similarities with principles and praxis from industrial product development and assembly system design, that is, a recommended building design process, guided by a correctly designed and utilized building program, since there will be a number of checkpoints ("gates"), defined beforehand (see Figure 14.3). These "gates" correspond to what, within the automotive industry, is denoted as product and process verifications.

This is a procedure that has been utilized within the building trade in Sweden for environmental aspects in building design and choice of materials as defined by Bergqvist and Rönn [16, 17] in accordance with the so-called environmental manual for the building sector [18].

The verification process that is sketched in Figure 14.3 is by no means unknown within the building trade, since in Sweden the responsible management, according to the law, is forced to participate with the employees during the reformation of premises. However, this is usually carried through as a restricted user (tenant) influence, verified only once during the building design process, namely, at the moment when the building permit is considered during the building phase. This dialogue is in most cases a matter of juridical interpretation of the work environment legislation [19] and not a broad, detailed, and long-term user (tenant) engagement as is described by Ahlin [20] and others. Accordingly, there are, in fact, elaborated routines and praxis available for a qualified user (tenant) influence and dialogue. Such formalized methods, in some cases providing possibilities for long-term user engagement, were used when the governmental authority (Kungliga Byggnadsstyrelsen) in Sweden was held responsible for governmental buildings.

To conclude, in the light of the authors' recent experiences and references to the literature mentioned above and elsewhere in this chapter, the problem area of user (tenant) participation within the building trade has not, during 20 years, been rectified. This is a fact even though knowledge as well as insights are easily accessible, as is evident by the references.

CONCLUSIONS

This chapter has described and recapitulated experiences from three projects regarding the design of public buildings that are in line with insights gained by the third author from the design of healthcare facilities. Three cases have been compared from the automotive industry, underlining vital facts concerning the building design process and the building trade's principles and praxis.

More detailed comparisons between the building trade and the automotive industry, as well as generalization, are called for to contrast two diametrically different positions, that is, the logic of the building trade and the logic of the automotive industry, respectively, each of which might be regarded as a representative extreme. In addition, if the argumentation were further detailed, the healthcare sector's facilities might be assumed to fall somewhere between these extremes.

On one hand, focusing on the materials flow aspects of "healthcare products," whatever this might be, the healthcare sector's building facilities are more connected to the automotive industry since, obviously, complex flows of "products" (various materials, different categories of employees, clients, etc.) are passing through the buildings. On the other hand, the university does not have such a discernible flow of "products" and definitely not the same demands for a detailed synchronization of various activities as the healthcare sector and the automotive industry. The eventual consequences of lack of fulfillment of the stipulated goals and agreements are not as obvious, nor do they demand immediate action from employees or management, as is the situation within the healthcare sector or the automotive industry.

Consequently, the impact of user (tenant) demands on the (physical)

Figure 14.4
**The Healthcare Sector's Building Facilities and Individual Competencies
versus the Automotive Industry and the University**

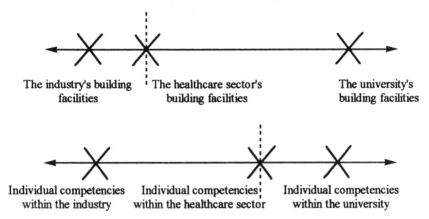

building facility might for the healthcare sector be assumed to resemble the conditions in the automotive industry rather than those at the university (Figure 14.4).

Figure 14.5 compares the healthcare sector characteristics and the automotive industry's and the university's characteristics regarding the aspects of product development, product specification, physical product, various users, and product life cycle aspects. This comparison might be debated as well as further examined in detail. However, it illuminates a procedure to condense the points of view and insights presented in this chapter.

However, if the point of convergence is the individual person's competence (operator in the automotive industry case), then the healthcare sector bears more resemblance to the university (the training and learning times required to become a professional is a matter of decades, depending on personal interests and ambitions). The automotive industry, on the other hand, has by tradition been striving for a delimited work content requiring low competence for most of the total work force (Figure 14.4). There are some evident exceptions, as mentioned above, but they are, in fact, neither fully recognized nor fully understood by most practitioners.

Note that this chapter does not refer to earlier principles and praxis, advocated by the automotive industry, such as extensive mechanized and automated equipment and automated guided vehicles systems (AGV systems). For example, these AGV systems were, according to the experiences of one of the authors, and still are, a technical fad not usually considered within the automotive industry to the same extent as was the

Figure 14.5
Company Healthcare and Automotive Sectors

	The Automotive Industry	The Healthcare Sector	The University
Some Product Development Aspects	Extensive long-term formalized product development work within the responsible organization.	Some long-term product development work within the responsible organization (e.g., research work).	Delimited formalized product development work within the responsible organization.
Some Product Specification Aspects	Defined far-reaching product specifications (e.g., product data included in a product structure) not communicated outside the responsible organization.	Some far-reaching product specifications exist which are communicated both inside and outside the responsible organization.	Lack of product specifications in the true sense.
Some Aspects on the Physical Product	Numerous deterministic standardized physical products (vehicles).	Many, both stochastic and deterministic, nonstandardized products (i.e., patients).	Some deterministic standardized virtual products (e.g., courses).
Some Aspects on Flows	Defined materials and product flows.	Complex mixed discernible materials flow.	Lack of discernible materials flow.
Some User Aspects	User of the product (i.e., customer) will define and care for.	User definition (i.e., patients or employees): extensive but heterogeneous.	User definitions on numerous "products" (i.e., pupils) are defined while other users (i.e., employees) are less carefully defined.
Some Product Life Cycle Aspects	Far-reaching product life cycle responsibilities.	Far-reaching product life cycle responsibilities.	Delimitation of product life cycle responsibilities.
General Comments	Private sector. Influenced by politics in the long-term perspective.	Public sector. Heavily influenced by politics in the short-term perspective.	Public sector. Heavily influenced by politics in the short-term perspective.

case 20 years ago when such a system was introduced at Östra Sjukhuset in Gothenburg.

The authors point to a "new," not yet fully crystallized manufacturing engineering concept, that is, principles and praxis where the so-called virtual artifact (product specification based on appropriate product data) is designed in congruence with the physical artifact (materials feeding technique, layouts, the choice of equipment and tools, etc.). This was the case for an assembly system design touched upon above.

The insights from industrial product development processes, on the other hand, also imply the general need for utilizing a more far-reaching product specification within the building trade, which in turn is applicable to the healthcare sector. It is far-reaching in the respect that it stretches from the beginning of the building design process to the user (tenant). This is a product specification that, as in the automotive industry, continuously reforms in relation to changes in environment and user (tenant) demands. The input for reformation has to be monitored and organized in quite a different way from today's practice in the building trade in order to create appropriate public buildings.

Industrial product development processes involve supplying a number of specific functions to answer user (tenant) demands, primarily in the form of building functions and secondary auxiliary functions. In accordance, the reasoning above concerning specifying the building facility might roughly be expressed as follows: to primarily furnish the specified functions of climate-controlled workplaces to a specified number of employees, which in turns requires lighting, electricity, external and internal communications, admitted separation of various defined categories of waste, permits for specified safety and security aspects, appropriate specified interfaces in relation to the user (tenant) in form of materials supply of defined items, telecommunications, and so on.

These functions ought to be continuously evaluated, preferably by defined methods during the (physical) building facility's total life, a procedure that must include the users (tenants) and employees' points of view. This might be a constructive future development of the umbrella term "facilities management."

But if practitioners and researchers accept the approach implied in the comparisons with industrial product development processes by specifying various building functions, they must also accept that this is complemented by determining the auxiliary services furnished by the property manager or other parties.

Figure 14.6 shows schematics of traditional procedure and recommended procedure—how to link the (physical) building facility to demands generated by the activities contained within the (physical) building facility.

Summing up, applying principles and praxis from industrial product

Figure 14.6
Traditional and Recommended Building Procedures

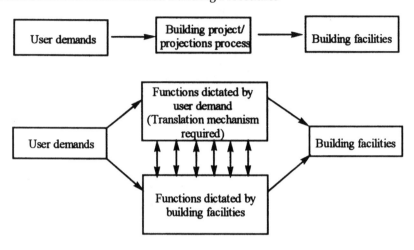

development processes and assembly system design to the building design process implies the need to shift focus from the physical building.
Thus building functions are transformed into a more abstract artifact (i.e.,
a so-called virtual artifact based on appropriate product data). This concept might be coined "conclusive product development." This is an artifact that is continuously changing—reforming in relation to various
changes in environment and user (tenant) demands. Input, which must
be monitored in quite another way than today, is praxis within the building trade, and not until then is it possible to create appropriate public
buildings. Accordingly, this will create a new platform for the "hospital
of the future."

NOTES

[1] Gasslander, J.-G., T. Engström, and Å. Wicklund, "The Industrial Product
    versus the Facility Product—A Framework for Crystallising the Healthcare
    Services of Tomorrow," 1st International Conference on The Hospital of the
    Future, Enschede, The Netherlands, 2001.
[2] Engström, T., D. Jonsson, and L. Medbo, "The Method of Successive Assem-
    bly System Design: Six Cases Studies within the Swedish Automotive In-
    dustry," in Gunarsekaran, A. (Ed.), *Agile Manufacturing: 21st Century
    Manufacturing Strategy* (New York: Elsevier Science Publishers, 2001).
[3] Engström, T., L.-G. Bergquist, J.-E. Gasslander, and R. Örtengren, "Brukar-
    medverkan vid planering, bygg och förvaltningsprocesser inom högskole-
    väsendet—Några erfarenheter, paralleller och reflektioner," in *Arbete
    människa miljö & Nordisk ergonomi* (in press).

[4] Dahlberg, J., "Bransch med miljardvinst," *Dagens Nyheter*, February 15, 2001, p. A11 (Swedish newspaper article).

[5] Medbo, L. "Materials Supply and Product Descriptions for Assembly System—Design and Operation," Ph.d. thesis, Department of Transportation and Logistics, Chalmers University of Technology, Göteborg, Sweden, 1999.

[6] Wätte, S., and P. Cassel, *Att använda kvalitetssystem inom byggsektorn. Vägvisare för beställare och arkitekter* (Stockholm: Sveriges Praktiserande Arkitekter, 1989).

[7] Bergqvist, L.-G., *Projektik och arbetsplatsens bruksform* (Göteborg: Institution för Form och Teknik, Chalmers Tekniska Högskola, 1994).

[8] Byggnadsstyrelsen, "Systemhandlingar kommentarer" Del 0–4, Byggnadsstyrelsens Rapporter 141, Byggnadsstyrelsen, Stockholm, 1979.

[9] Lundholm, A.-M., "Kris hotar Naturhistoriska riksmuseet. 40 medarbetare kan få sluta. Regeringen kompenserar inte inflation i. Hyran tar halva anslaget," *Svenska Daglandet*, June 11, 1996, p. 15

[10] Muther, R., *Systematic Layout Planning* (Boston: Planning Industrial Education Institute, 1961).

[11] Statens Arbetsmiljönämnd, "Personalmedverkan vid lokalplanering," SAN rapport, Statens Arbetsmiljönämnd, Stockholm, 1979.

[12] Carlsson, T. "Billigt åskskydd fungerar inte—Varje blixtnedslag skadar hundratals elektroniska apparater," *Ny Teknik*, No. 32, 2000, p. 20.

[13] IVA, *Produktframtagning i fokus—En spegling av produkt- och processutveckling hos ett verkstadsföretag och ett byggföretag* (Stockholm: Kungliga Ingenjörsvetenskapsakademin [IVA], 1998).

[14] SOU, "Sammanfattning och förslag. Särtryck av Byggkostnadsdelegationens Slutbetänkande," *Byggkostnadsdelegationen*, 44, 2000.

[15] Sundsvik, L., J. Höjer, and K. Mellander, in "Byggprocesser," *Byggforskningsrådet* (Stockholm: T2D, 1983).

[16] Bergqvist, L.-G., and M. Rönn, "En ny agenda för projektering. Erfarenheter av metodstudie 1:2," Form och Teknik, Chalmers Tekniska Högskola, Göteborg, Sweden, 1999.

[17] Bergqvist, L.-G., and M. Rönn, "En ny agenda för projektering. Metod för miljöstyrning i byggprojekt 2—Södermalmshemmet," Form och Teknik, Chalmers Tekniska Högskola, Göteborg, Sweden, 2000.

[18] Miljöstiftelsen för Byggsektorn, "Miljömanualen för Byggsektorn," Miljöstiftelsen för Byggsektorn, 1989.

[19] Bergqvist, L.-G., M. Käppi, M. Rönn, and D. Töllborg, "Skyddsombud överklagar," Studentlitteratur, 1989.

[20] Ahlin, J., "Mönsterpråket för arbetsmiljöplanering," in *Avdelningen för Projekteringsmetodik* (Stockholm: Kungliga Tekniska Högskolan, 1980).

Chapter 15

The Dynamic Hospital (Building) of the Future

*Corina M. J. Schols, Bert-Jan Grevink,
and Annette Molkenboer-Hamming*

INTRODUCTION

This chapter presents a conceptual view of developments in the Dutch healthcare system that may change the structure of health care and the location of hospital functions. The chapter starts with a view of future health care. Because of the changing view of health and health care, we expect the demand for hospital functions and their locations to change. Therefore, a formula for the dispersion of hospital functions is introduced. On the basis of this formula, developments in both the demand side and the supply side of hospital health care are described. As these developments seem to lead to the concentration of specialized health care on the one hand and decentralization of more basic health care on the other hand, the hospital of the future will need buildings and facilities at more than one location. These different locations are described and, finally, a view is given of how the required flexibility and expandability of hospital buildings can be handled.

A VIEW OF FUTURE HEALTH CARE

In order to develop a conceptual view of future hospital buildings, it is necessary to think first about future health care in general and hospital health care in particular.

The way people feel about health and health care is changing. In the future, we expect people to get healthier and to live longer. Figure 15.1 shows the "healthline" of a healthy person born today and in the future. Life expectancy is still rising, mainly because of a decline in mortality of

Figure 15.1
A View of Future Health Care

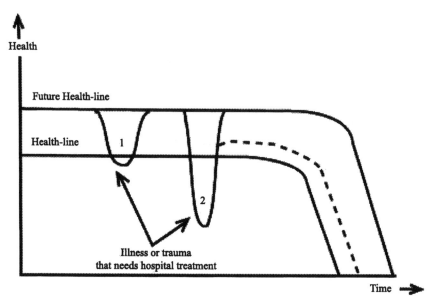

heart diseases and cancer. Compared to the clearly unhealthy years, the amount of healthy and slightly unhealthy years will grow during one's lifetime [1]. According to Vos, Dutch citizens know a lot and want a lot but are also concerned about their state of health [1]. People no longer think that health is something to strive for. Health has become a norm. They want to stay as healthy as possible during their whole life.

In order to stay healthy as long as possible, we have to live healthy, eat healthy, exercise, and so forth. In a word, we have to maintain our minds and bodies continuously in order to keep at a certain level of health. This can be called "preventive maintenance" or "preventive health care." However, during our lives, illness or trauma can occur, which causes us to deviate from our initial healthline [2]. In these cases, we need "corrective maintenance"—an intervention or other kind of hospital treatment—in order to stay alive and get healthy again. For smaller problems and corrections, we go see a general practitioner (GP), and for recovery from illness or trauma we are looked after in nursing homes or are supported by home care. And sometimes we are not able to get back to our initial level of health but have to live at a lower level of health.

Today's medicine is almost entirely about these acute deviations. Developments in medical technology (e.g., nanotechnology) will make it possible to treat diseases and trauma that cannot be treated today. Therefore, it will become possible to recover from deeper dips in the healthline. However, most health and disease happens over a lifetime, not in a moment of crisis. Trauma happens in a moment—a gunshot, a car wreck. But even trauma is usually a result of lifestyles, habits, addictions, and environments that extend over years and decades. The most effective health care is therefore framed by long-term relationships [2].

This call for long-term relationships will be supported by developments in, for example, the Human Genome Project. The Human Genome Project may isolate the genetic roots of many human diseases and make it possible to screen mass populations. As the slope of individual healthlines becomes more predictable, it will become possible to prevent (through diet, gene substitution, or other special therapies) specific diseases that individuals are likely to develop. It will also be possible to intervene earlier in cases of predictable diseases [3]. This might prevent large dips in people's healthlines.

Hospitals today are focusing on sick care in order to restore people to health. In the future, the focus of health care will be on supporting people's healthlines during their whole life, not just in cases of illness or trauma. Maintaining health or preventing illness will become more important. Therefore, the hospital, which essentially provides sick care, will not be the natural driver of the "health chain."

The GP will be a more natural driver but, as with hospitals, we consult a GP when we are ill. In our view, prevention will be the main aspect of future health care, and therefore a new kind of medical function—preventive health care—will probably appear in the near future. Perhaps it is possible to compare this new function with dental care. We go to a dentist for a checkup every six months, even when our teeth do not hurt. We do this as prevention, to keep our teeth healthy. The dentist supports us with information about how to prevent getting cavities, and in case we do get a cavity, it is treated by the dentist. If there are more serious problems, the dentist refers us to a dental surgeon.

Because of the changing view of health and health care, the demand for hospital functions will change. Important developments include increased life expectancy, health becoming a norm, and health care moving from treatment to prevention and intervention. These developments influence the attitude of the patient toward health care and therefore toward the location of healthcare delivery. Furthermore, due to developments in medical technology and information and communication technology, the supply of hospital functions will change. We expect these changes to have an impact on the dispersion of hospital functions in the future.

DISPERSION OF HOSPITAL FUNCTIONS

Hospitals can be characterized as service organizations. Service organizations are essentially facilitating systems that enable the clients to realize their own goals in direct interaction with the service provider. In order to provide adequate service, these organizations need facilities as much as possible in the vicinity of their clients. So, like other service organizations, one would expect hospital organizations to have facilities in the vicinity of their patients. However, dispersion of hospital functions nowadays is limited. Most hospital buildings are huge and complex and accommodate many different and sometimes very specialized functions. The ongoing mergers between Dutch hospitals, for example, do not seem to lead to more dispersion but, on the contrary, to even more concentrated functions.

Merging Hospitals

Presently, merging seems to be an attractive strategy for Dutch hospitals. Together, the merged hospitals expect to be more capable of providing high-quality health care and be better prepared for future developments. Now that the merged hospitals have at their disposal buildings at different locations, one would expect the hospitals—as service organizations—to use these different locations to provide healthcare services closer to their patients. However, many hospitals want to concentrate all their functions in one building or at least on the same site. Concentration of services in the short term is seldom possible, so the "more location" situation is seen as a temporary inconvenience. Recent experiences with merged hospitals show that most people working in hospitals feel they should be housed at the "head location" that accommodates the clinic and the intensive care unit. This does not only involve specialists who want their preclinical activities at this location but also medical support functions, like the pharmacy, laboratories, and so forth.

For a long time, it was indeed very profitable for specialists to work together at one hospital location. Due to the ongoing developments in medical science and technology, the increasing costs of medical equipment, and the advantages of teamwork, medical specialists settled down in hospitals. However, nowadays, or at least in the near future, it is no longer necessary to be in each other's direct neighborhood to take advantage of these benefits. Furthermore, patients increasingly ask for hospital services within a limited distance of home or work.

A Theoretical Approach of Hospital Dispersion

In deciding about the measure of dispersion of functions one always has to think about the match between the request for dispersion on the one hand and the possibilities for dispersion on the other hand. This can be represented as follows:

The first formula represents the request for dispersion of hospital functions by the patient (the demand side). It is determined by the amount of interventions needed and by the impact the intervention has on the patient. When the amount of interventions needed becomes higher or the impact of the intervention becomes lower, the request for dispersion of hospital functions will grow.

The second formula represents the possibility of dispersion of hospital functions (the supply side). The decentralization of hospital functions is limited by the availability of technology, skilled professionals, and funds. The governmental control of Dutch hospital health care also plays a role in the limitation of decentralization of hospital functions.

Future developments in society, demographics, and technology—some of which are already visible nowadays—will influence the demand and supply side of this formula and therefore the level at which they will match. These developments and their expected impact on the dispersion of hospital functions are described in the following sections.

The Request for Dispersion of Hospital Functions

Treatments that take place with a high frequency and a low impact on the patient can be called "basic health care." For this kind of care, the request for dispersion is high. For example, the recent commotion about cutting back the functions in the hospitals in Oldenzaal and Zierikzee (small Dutch towns) shows clearly that people don't want to travel long distances for basic health care. People want to be treated near their homes for the interventions or treatments that are more routine. However, when the impact of an intervention is higher and more specialized care and cure is necessary, people are more willing to travel to a hospital location. These interventions and treatments can therefore be concentrated. This is also necessary in order to provide a higher quality of specialized health care and to enable medical specialists to increase their knowledge in their specific field.

The amount of interventions or treatments needed and the impact they have on the patient is influenced by technological developments, by medical developments, the number of inhabitants, and the constitution of the population. When the amount of interventions or treatments of a certain kind rises, the experience with these interventions grows. The Dutch elderly of the future (who will be most in need of health care) will probably be in a relatively better economic position. They will consider health to be most important, and therefore they will want to be able to "buy" health(care) whenever possible, and increasingly they will demand that basic health care be provided near their homes. As funds, skilled people, and necessary technology for basic health care become more available, it will be easier to decentralize these kinds of hospital functions. Therefore, it can be expected that the low impact interventions and treatments will move out of the acute-care hospital and will get dispersed through the region.

The Possibility of Dispersion of Hospital Functions

Technology is one of the important determinants of the possibilities in health care. One of the most recent examples of the impact technology can have on providing health care is the possibility of performing operations at a distance. As better use is made of this new technology and as hospitals become more experienced with it, the more common it becomes. In the future, operating at a distance may even become part of basic health care. This can also be the case for future developments we don't yet even know.

Traditionally, the entire treatment given to any individual patient has tended to be fragmented. Patients have been passed across a variety of barriers from primary to secondary and secondary to tertiary care. Even within each sector of the healthcare service, particularly in the secondary care sector, a number of minor "baton changes" were occurring. Consider how many times an individual patient is asked his or her name and address and how many times records are mislaid or dispersed. This is all the result of too much emphasis on designing systems for the convenience of the provider, rather than around the needs of the user [4].

Nowadays, the emphasis on the provider becomes less important due to a growing focus on the patient. This is shown by the efforts to develop an EPR (electronic patient record). The EPR makes it easier to communicate within each sector of the service as well as between the different sectors. Furthermore, the primary, secondary, and tertiary sectors are working together more and more. They become partners in the "health chain" in order to support the environment with all kinds of needed health care. This is extremely important, as the focus of health care will change from acute episodes to long-term health care.

Next to the changing focus in health care, there are also developments in information and communications technology, a growing focus on outcomes management, and the introduction of new management strategies. These will have an enormous impact on how health care will be provided in the future.

In the near future, a shortage of doctors, specialists, and nurses is expected in the Netherlands. As a matter of fact, this is already the case, and it is not expected that this shortage will soon be addressed. Therefore, it is necessary to distinguish between interventions and treatments that are necessarily reserved for medical specialists and treatments that can be done by people with different skills. Presently, we already see that GPs or nurses are performing treatments previously done by medical specialists. Developments in ICT (Information and Communication Technology) will make it possible to provide health care independent of time and place. Because of the ongoing developments in medical technology, this technology will become cheaper and easier to handle and therefore more available. The example of the GP who is using X-ray technology proves that this is already happening.

Conclusion

Because of the desired focus on the patient, the hospital will become a real service organization that focuses on interventions and specialized treatments. The necessary match between supply and demand of hospital health care will take place at two different levels. One is the level of "basic care and cure," which needs to be provided in proximity to the patients and the other is the level of the "acute and specialized care and cure," which needs to be concentrated in order to efficiently use scarce supplies of technology and skilled professionals.

Because of the developments listed above, the definition of basic care will change over time. More and more interventions will be considered basic care, hence the impact of the intervention on the patient will become lower. The low-impact interventions will become more frequent and more predictable. This trend is shown in the ongoing transfer of clinical treatments to preclinical treatments or same-day surgery. Very importantly, as elderly people, who are the most in need of health care, are willing to pay for health care, they will require it to be provided in their own neighborhood.

On the other hand, the ongoing developments in medical technology will lead to more capabilities in medical care. People who can't be treated nowadays will be treated in the future. Interventions with a bigger impact on the patient will become possible. This kind of hospital care needs to be concentrated in order to make efficient use of the more specialized skills, available technology, and funds. Centralization of these hospital functions is not a problem, as the need for these kinds of interventions is much lower, while the impact on the patient is very high.

Hospitals will be increasingly able to disperse some of their functions if sufficient technology, skilled professionals, and funds are available. Dutch health care has mostly been financed and directed by the government. Hospitals have always depended on the approval of the government for funds. Now that the Dutch government is continually stepping down, hospitals will have more influence on the use of funds. In our view, the changing attitude of the government, along with the described changes in supply and demand of health care, will lead to a few specialized intervention centers and a lot of healthcare service centers closer to the patient. These specialized intervention centers will be centers of expertise. Functions that are now part of the specialized intervention

Figure 15.2
Dispersion of Hospital Functions

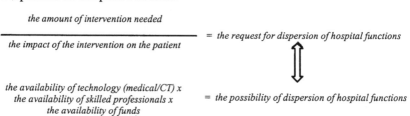

the amount of intervention needed
———————————————————————— = *the request for dispersion of hospital functions*
the impact of the intervention on the patient

⇕

the availability of technology (medical/CT) x
the availability of skilled professionals x   = *the possibility of dispersion of hospital functions*
the availability of funds

center will become part of the healthcare service center, while the functions at the specialized intervention center will continually change due to ongoing technological developments. In the future, this dynamic process will be characteristic of hospital organizations.

THE DYNAMIC HOSPITAL BUILDINGS OF THE FUTURE

In the future, concentration will not be required by patients and will no longer be necessary for cooperation of specialists. It will become attractive to concentrate only very specific hospital functions, while bringing more common hospital functions closer to the patient.

This will not only influence the hospital organization and its processes. Concentration and dispersion of hospital functions will also influence the buildings and other facilities required to support these continually changing hospital functions. The hospital will need facilities at several locations—smaller facilities at several locations in the region (health service centers) to accommodate the dispersed functions and bigger facilities at an easily accessible location to accommodate the concentrated functions. Since functions will continually transfer to the decentralized health service centers as new functions enter the concentrated intervention center, flexibility in the buildings at both centers is a necessity (see Figure 15.2).

Thus, the changing view of the Dutch government, in which hospital buildings are considered hospital affairs rather than governmental affairs, creates many opportunities. It is time to consider buildings and other facilities as a means of production. Clearly, it won't be possible to optimize the capacity of buildings that must last about 40 years. After all, treatments that take place at the centralized intervention center at $t = 0$ will take place at the satellites at $t = x$. When planning new facilities it is not possible to be certain about x. So, neither the precise timing of the health service center expansion nor the necessary adaptations are predictable. At the same time, it is not possible to predict the necessary alterations of the concentrated buildings.

However, the request for flexibility and expandability in hospital buildings is not new. For example, the research of Stolwijk [5] and Mens and Tijhuis [6] ascertained that Dutch hospitals are continually adapting and expanding their buildings. "Because of the complexity of hospital organizations and the diversity in a lot of factors such as operations, functions, cooperation, and development, the size of alterations and expansions is very varied" [5].

The dynamics of concentration and decentralization and the necessity of flexibility and expandability have shaped our view on the hospital buildings of the future.

The Health Service Centers

The health service centers provide "basic health care" that varies from preclinical care and diagnostic functions to day surgery and day care and, in some cases, short stay. These "satellite" functions will still be hospital functions, but will be combined with other healthcare services in order to support people in maintaining their healthlines. It is possible to think about combinations with GPs, physiotherapists, psychologists, dieticians, pharmacies, dentists, homeopaths, and so on. But, more commercially oriented functions such as opticians, suppliers of hearing aids, sporting schools, swimming pools, and drugstores belong to the optional combinations. For healthcare-oriented organizations like health insurers and home care organizations, these healthcare service centers can also become attractive residences.

The amount of services delivered at the several centers depends on the request for dispersion and the possibility of dispersion. With regard to hospital functions, there will be comparatively smaller centers with mainly preclinical and diagnostic functions and fewer centers that also have same-day surgery or day care. In order to provide short stay, it will be necessary to add such services as a nursing home.

However, as technological developments accumulate, the increase and alterations of the dispersed functions will be quite common. Therefore, it might perhaps be best to rent space at healthcare service centers to accommodate the dispersed functions of the hospital.

The Specialized Intervention Center

With regard to the facilities at the intervention center, it is difficult to predict future technological developments. What kind of treatments will become possible in the future and what kind of technology (e.g., medical equipment) will this require? Therefore, the facilities needed to support the processes at this center will have to deal with continuous change.

When activities expand, it should be possible to extend buildings as well as equipment and installations easily.

As flexibility and expandability are necessary conditions for most hospital functions, it does not seem advisable to accommodate all functions in the same building. First, the different functions need very different facilities, floor area, equipment, and installations. Therefore, it is not easy to exchange functions. This is visible today, as many hospitals scale back the number of beds and expand their preclinical activities. The sections used for clinical care are becoming obsolete but cannot easily be used for preclinical activities. Secondly, adaptations in buildings and installations cause much inconvenience and will sometimes even disrupt the hospital processes. When all functions are in the same building, they will be disrupted every time alterations occur. Therefore, developing different buildings with a specific purpose will become attractive. These different buildings and their surroundings can be shaped like a university campus.

The Idea of a Campus

The different hospital functions with different facilities need to be accommodated in different buildings. We can think of a diagnostic building, a building for preclinical services, a building for day surgery and day care, a building for special medical treatment and intensive care, a laboratory building, a logistic center, an office building, and an educational/scientific building. Facilities like restaurants and shops already exist in most hospitals. Furthermore, the site and its buildings should be attractive to patients, as it is well known that the surroundings influence people's mind and health.

All the shared facilities should be centrally located and widely accessible. For meetings or at meal times, users of the hospital will therefore have to go to the central facilities, which will facilitate contact between the different specialists and hospital employees. A highly modern information and communication infrastructure (which will even be cordless in part) should be available in order to provide rapid exchange of knowledge on the campus as well as with the outside world.

Developing different buildings with a specific purpose and at a specific location will be more flexible and more durable. When activities expand, it will be possible to extend buildings, equipment, and installations more easily, without disturbing all other hospital functions. Alternatively, when the buildings cannot satisfy the hospital needs anymore, it will be possible to change them into other functions. For example, a building for clinical care of patients essentially has a hotel function and administrative hospital function that are actually accommodated in office facilities. Preclinical facilities are very useful as apartments, as the design for reusing the former hospital at the Gedempte Burgwal in The Hague shows [7]. Reusing these facilities as apartments for elderly people who need certain kinds of care could be attractive for both the hospital and the possible inhabitants.

Another attractive strategy can be to plan these buildings so they already have both hospital and other functions. Building a hotel and using it partly for clinical care of patients while renting out the other part to a commercial hotel can be a very flexible solution. When fewer clinical beds are needed, a larger part of the hotel will be rented out, and vice versa. This kind of flexibility is also possible with the office functions, the educational functions, and the central facilities. It might also be attractive—because of economies of scale—to combine laboratory functions with other hospitals or other organizations.

NOTES

[1] Vos, P., "De trend, de traditie en de turbulentie: Turbulentie-analyse Nederlandse gezondheidszorg," *Raad voor de volksgezondheid en zorg* (Amsterdam: Zoetermeer, November 1999).

[2] Flower, J., and P. Guillaume, *The Healthcare Team of the Future*, www. healthcentral.com/columnists, December 7, 2000.

[3] Flower, J., *The Future of Health Care: Encyclopedia of the Future* (New York: Macmillan, 1996).

[4] Nugent, R., "Shaping the Future," *Hospital Development*, 26–27, 1995, 11–12.

[5] Stolwijk, W. Q., *Flexibiliteit in ziekenhuisbouw*; Universiteit Delft (Arnhem: Proefschrift Technische Universiteit Delft, 1987).

[6] Mens, N., and A. Tijhuis, *De architectuur van het ziekenhuis* (Rotterdam: NAI Uitgevers, 1999).

[7] De Ridder and Schnater Architecten, www.res.box.nl/gb97/gb97.htm, Rotterdam.

Suggested Readings

This is a list of suggested readings on topics related to the Hospital of the Future. It is by no means an exhaustive list. Rather, it contains selected works in the intersection between healthcare delivery, management, and technology. Some of these works are cited in the preceding chapters.

This list of suggested readings is aimed at researchers, students, and practitioners who are interested in expanding their horizons beyond this book. The variety of topics covered by the suggested readings is illustrative of the complexity of the area of the Hospital of the Future. It is not only a multidisciplinary area for research and practice, but also includes subareas of interfaces among the disciplines. Even with the enclosed list of readings, we have just begun to scratch the surface of this challenging and highly intricate topic of the Hospital of the Future and the various aspects of future healthcare delivery.

Allison, S., and K. McLaughlin-Renpenning, *Nursing Administration in the 21st Century* (Thousand Oaks, CA: Sage Publications, 1998).

Altman, S., U. Reinhardt, and A. Shields (Eds.), *The Future U.S. Healthcare System: Who Will Care for the Poor and Uninsured?* (Chicago: Health Administration Press, 1998).

Armstrong, C., *AHA Guide to Computerized Physician Order Entry Systems* (Chicago: American Hospital Association Press, 2000).

Brook, R. H., C. J. Kamberg, and E. A. McGlynn, "Health System Reform and Quality," *Journal of the American Medical Association*, 276(6), 1996, 476–480.

Brown, M., *Integrated Healthcare Delivery* (Frederick, MD: Aspen Publishers, 1996).

Clare, M., D. Sargent, R. Moxley, and T. Forthman, "Reducing Health Care Delivery Costs Using Clinical Paths: A Case Study on Improving Hospital Profitability," *Journal of Health Care Finance*, 21(3), 1995, 48–58.

Coddington, D., and K. Moore, *Capitalizing Medical Groups: Positioning Physicians for the Future* (New York: McGraw-Hill, 1997).

Coddington, D., K. Moore, and E. Fischer, *Strategies for the New Health Care Marketplace: Managing the Convergence of Consumerism and Technology* (San Francisco: Jossey-Bass, 2001).

Coile, R., *The New Hospital: Future Strategies for a Changing Industry* (Gaithersburg, MD: Aspen Publishers, 1986).

Cooper, R., and R. Layard (Eds.), *What the Future Holds* (Boston: MIT Press, 2002).

Dranove, D., *The Economic Evolution of American Health Care* (Princeton, NJ: Princeton University Press, 2000).

Edwards, T., and T. Mayer, *Urgent Care Medicine* (New York: McGraw-Hill, 2002).

Fisher, G., *Health Care and Insurance: Distortions Imposed on the Medical System by Its Financing* (New York: Lightning Source, 2001).

Flower, J., *The Future of Healthcare: Encyclopedia of the Future* (New York: Macmillan, 1996).

Forman, P. N., "Information Needs of Physicians," *Journal of the American Society of Information Sciences*, 46(10), 1995, 729–736.

Fukuyama, F., *Our Posthuman Future: Consequences of the Biotechnology Revolution* (New York: Farrar, Strauss & Giroux, 2002).

Fulop, N., P. Allen, A. Clarke, and N. Black, *Studying the Organization and Delivery of Health Services: Research Methods* (London: Routledge, 2001).

Gaucher, E., and R. Coffey, *Breakthrough Performance: Accelerating the Transformation of Healthcare Organizations* (San Francisco: Jossey-Bass, 2000).

Geisler, E., and O. Heller, *Managing Technology in Healthcare* (Boston: Kluwer Academic Publishers, 1996).

Geisler, E., and O. Heller, *Management of Medical Technology: Theory, Practice, and Cases* (Boston: Kluwer Academic Publishers, 1998).

Goldman, S., and C. Graham, *Agility in Health Care: Strategies for Mastering Turbulent Markets* (San Francisco: Jossey-Bass, 1998).

Goldstein, D., *e-Healthcare: Harness the Power of Internet e-Commerce & e-Care* (Frederick, MD: Aspen Publishers, 2000).

Goodman, J., and C. Vernon, *The Heart Hospital: A Reality of the Future* (New York: John Goodman & Associates, 1997).

Grbich, C., *Qualitative Research in Health* (Thousand Oaks, CA: Sage Publications, 1998).

Greene, J., *Hospitals and Healthcare Systems of the Future* (Washington, DC: American Institute of Architects Press, 1996).

Grutter, R. (Ed.), *Knowledge Media in Healthcare: Opportunities and Challenges* (Hershey, PA: Idea Group Publishing, 2002).

Harrison, A., and S. Prentice, *Hospital Policy in the United Kingdom: Its Development, Its Future* (London: Transaction Publishing, 1997).

Heathfield, H., and G. Louw, "New Challenges for Clinical Informatics: Knowledge Management Tools," *Health Informatics Journal* 5, 1999, 67–73.

Jennings, M., *Health Care Strategy for Uncertain Times* (San Francisco: Jossey-Bass, 2000).

Kleinke, J., *Oxymorons: The Myth of a U.S. Health Care System* (San Francisco: Jossey-Bass, 2001).

Lerman, D. (Ed.), *Home Care: Positioning the Hospital for the Future* (Chicago: American Hospital Publishing, 1987).

Lundberg, G., *Severed Trust: Why American Medicine Hasn't Been Fixed* (New York: Basic Books, 2001).

Maheu, M., P. Whitten, and A. Allen, *E-Health, Telehealth, and Telemedicine: A Guide to Startup and Success* (San Francisco: Jossey-Bass, 2001).

Marsh, A. (Ed.), *Advanced Infrastructures for Future Healthcare* (New York: IOS Press, 2001).

Nash, D., M. Manfredi, B. Bozarth, and S. Howell, *Connecting with the New Healthcare Consumer: Defining Your Strategy* (Frederick, MD: Aspen Publishers, 2001).

Nesmith, E., *Health Care Architecture: Designs for the Future* (Washington, DC: American Institute of Architects, 1995).

Orlikoff, J., and M. Toffen, *The Future of Healthcare Governance: Redesigning Boards for a New Era* (Chicago: American Hospital Publishing, 1996).

Persily, N. (Ed.), *Eldercare: Positioning Your Hospital for the Future* (Chicago: American Hospital Publishing, 1991).

Preker, A., and A. Harding (Eds.), *Hospital Reform: Innovations in Health Care* (Washington, DC: The World Bank, 2002).

Sells, D., *Security in the Healthcare Environment* (Frederick, MD: Aspen Publishers, 2000).

Shelton, P., *Measuring and Improving Patient Satisfaction* (Frederick, MD: Aspen Publishers, 2000).

Sheng, O. R., "Decision Support for Health Care in a New Information Age," *Decision Support Systems*, 30(2), 2000, 101–103.

Shi, L., and D. Singh, *Delivering Health Care in America: A Systems Approach*, 2nd ed. (Frederick, MD: Aspen Publishers, 2000).

Slack, W., *Cybermedicine: How Computing Empowers Doctors and Patients for Better Care* (San Francisco: Jossey-Bass, 2001).

Smith, D., and T. Sullivan, *Nursing 2020: A Study of the Future of Hospital-Based Nursing* (Washington, DC: National League Press, 1988).

Snook, D., *Hospitals: What They Are and How They Work*, 2nd ed. (Frederick, MD: Aspen Publishers, 1999).

Sunseri, R., and A. Solovy, *Leadership Report: Key Issues Shaping the Future of Health Care* (Chicago: American Hospital Publishing, 1999).

Taylor-Moss, M., *Re-engineering of Operative and Invasive Services: Preparing for the Capitated Dollar* (Frederick, MD: Aspen Publishers, 1996).

Turnbull, J., and C. Beacock, *Managing and Leading Innovation Health Care* (New York: W. B. Saunders Company, 2002).

Vegoda, P., *Integrating the Health Care Enterprise* (New York: HIMSS Publications, 2001).

Weed, L. L., "New Connections Between Medical Knowledge and Patient Care," *British Medical Journal*, 315, 1997, 231–235.

Wolper, L., *Health Care Administration: Planning, Implementing, and Managing Organized Delivery Systems*, 3rd ed. (Frederick, MD: Aspen Publishers, 1999).

World Market Research Center, *Hospital Engineering and Facility Management* (London: International Federation of Hospital Engineering, 2002).

Zey, M., *The Future Factor: The Five Forces Transforming Our Lives and Shaping Human Destiny* (New York: McGraw-Hill Professional Publishing, 2000).

Index

About the Editors and Contributors

ELIEZER GEISLER is Professor of Organizational Behavior at Stuart Graduate School of Business, Illinois Institute of Technology. Professor Geisler is the author of over 80 papers in scientific journals and six books. He is associate editor of the *International Journal of Healthcare Technology and Management* and the editor of a series of special issues for the *International Journal of Technology Management*. Professor Geisler was also co-editor of a book series on *Management of Medical Technology* for Kluwer Academic Publishers. His recent books are *The Metrics of Science and Technology* (Quorum Books, 2000) and *Creating Value with Science and Technology* (Quorum Books, 2001).

Professor Geisler's current areas of research include the management of medical technology (MMT) and the evaluation and measurement of science and technology. He is a member of the Academy of Management and a senior member of the Institute of Electrical and Electronic Engineers.

KOOS KRABBENDAM is Professor of Operations Management in the School of Management Studies at the University of Twente, The Netherlands, where he also served as dean from 1993 until 1999. He has held several positions in the scientific community and is a member of the board of supervisors of TSM Business School. Since 1997 he is visiting professor at the Hunan International Business School, People's Republic of China. At present he is involved in research in healthcare technology and management.

ROEL W. SCHURING is Associate Professor of "Management of Health Care Organizations" in the University of Twente. He spent the first years of his research career studying manufacturing organizations and learned how technology, organizational arrangements, and individuals each contribute in their own way to the reality of operational processes. The complexity of organizations and operational processes in the healthcare sector is currently the empirical field to study the process modeling of organizations. The introduction of new technologies and information technology are currently his areas of interest. Schuring has published in journals such as the *International Journal of Operations* and *Technology Management*.

LAURENCE ALPAY is with the Klinishe Informatiekunde, Leiden University Medical Center, Leiden, The Netherlands.

ALEX APPLEBY is with the Center for Business Excellence, University of Northumbria, United Kingdom.

CHRISTOPHER M. BARLOW is with the Stuart Graduate School of Business, Illinois Institute of Technology, Chicago, Illinois.

LARS GÖRAN BERGQVIST is with the Department of Building Design, Chalmers University of Technology, Sweden.

HANS K. C. BLOO is with Roessingh Research and Development, B.V., Enschede, The Netherlands.

CECILIA CABELLO is with the Superior Council for Scientific Research (CSIC), Comparative Policy and Politics Unit, Madrid, Spain.

AMERICO CICCHETTI is with the Program in Health Economics and Management at the A. Gemelli School of Medicine of the Università Cattolica del Sacro Cuore, Rome, Italy.

MAXINE CONNER is with the Northern and Yorkshire Region of the National Health System Learning Alliance, Birmingham, United Kingdom.

CAROL DAVIES is Senior Research Fellow with the Center for Health Services Studies, University of Warwick, United Kingdom.

GRAYDON DAVISON is with the Incite Research Center, University of Western Sydney, Australia.

RENNEE DOOYEWEERD is a doctoral candidate at the Department of Healthcare and Management, University of Twente, The Netherlands.

TOMAS ENGSTRÖM is Associate Professor and head of the Materials Handling Research Group at Chalmers University of Technology, Sweden.

JOHN FITZGIBBON is with the Triple G Corporation, Markham, Ontario, Canada.

JAN-ERIK GASSLANDER is research leader at Chalmers University, Department of Transportation and Logistics, and Industrial Relations Officer at Malmo University, Sweden.

BERT-JAN GREVINK is with Pieterse Terwel Grevink Advies B.V., The Netherlands.

PAUL HYLAND is with Central Queensland University, Australia.

ROB F. M. KLEISSEN is with the Faculty of Technology and Management, Institute for Health Care Technology and Management, University of Twente, The Netherlands.

UIJA LÄMSÄ is a doctoral student at the University of Oulu in Finland.

CRAIG A. LEHMANN is Dean of Health Technology and Management, State University of New York at Stony Brook.

ANNETTE MOLKENBOER-HAMMING is with Pieterse Terwel Grevink Advies B.V., The Netherlands.

LUIS SANZ-MENENDEZ is with the Training and Education Group, Spanish Policy Research in Innovation and Technology, CSIC, Madrid, Spain.

TAINA SAVOLAINEN is Professor of Quality Management, Helsinki University of Technology, Lahti, Finland.

CORINA M. J. SCHOLS is with Pieterse Terwel Grevink Advies B.V., The Netherlands.

WIM H. VAN HARTEN is with the Roessingh Center for Rehabilitation, Enschede, The Netherlands.

PIETER VIERHOUT is surgeon and traumatologist at the Medisch Spectrum Twente Teaching Hospital in Enschede, The Netherlands. He is also Chair of the Department of Surgery at Medisch Spectrum Hospital. In

1999 he was appointed Professor of Health Care and Management at the University of Twente. In 2001 Dr. Vierhout was elected President of the Board of the Netherlands Association of Surgeons.

PAUL WALLEY is Lecturer in Operations Management at Warwick Business School, United Kingdom.

ÅKE WIKLUND is Professor of Design of Hospitals and Health Care, School of Architecture, Chalmers University of Technology, Sweden.